CW00504948

IN SUSPICIOUS
CIRCUMSTANCES

IN SUSPICIOUS CIRCUMSTANCES

Memories of a
NORTHAMPTONSHIRE
Police Surgeon

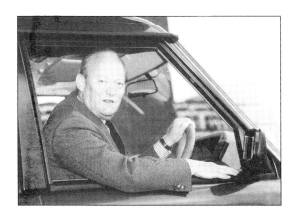

Hugh de la Haye Davies

COUNTRYSIDE BOOKS
NEWBURY, BERKSHIRE

First published 1998
© Hugh de la Haye Davies 1998

COUNTRYSIDE BOOKS
3 Catherine Road
Newbury, Berkshire

ISBN 1 85306 546 3

Produced through MRM Associates Ltd., Reading
Printed by J. W. Arrowsmith Ltd., Bristol

This book is dedicated to Dr Judith Thomas, Police Surgeon, Northamptonshire Police, who died of breast cancer at the age of 34 on the 10th January 1998. 'Popular with police and prisoners alike, compassionate and caring with victims of crime, her gentle and infectious smile would be guaranteed to defuse any awkward situation, calm the most obstreperous prisoner, and comfort a nervous child or adult victim.'

CONTENTS

INTRODUCTION

For 37 years I worked closely with the Northamptonshire Police, starting as an assistant to a general practice in Northampton that provided medical services to the County Constabulary and becoming in time Principal Police Surgeon.

In those early days I was mainly concerned with the health of the officers and in giving advice to the Chief Constable on medical matters, but I was also called in when a police officer needed the assistance of a doctor in the execution of his duties. This covered a multitude of sins under the heading of what today falls into the discipline of clinical forensic medicine. In 1958, however, it was not a heavy workload and usually included such relatively trivial matters as examining drivers to confirm whether or not they were 'drunk in charge', and the occasional dead body to confirm that there was no prima facie evidence of foul play.

At that time general practice in a country market town was a very attractive and rewarding occupation. Life was lived at a much slower pace and the country was at last beginning to get back to normal after the years of austerity following the end of the Second World War. However, I gradually found myself doing more police work, on a national as well as local level, as crime increased. This was in line with both the population growth of the county and the national increase in crime (especially in violent crime) since the early 1960s. Experience gained from general practice and from working as a clinical assistant in the Ear, Nose and Throat department of Northampton General Hospital, provided me with a good grounding on which to build my forensic expertise. Eventually, after 24 years in the NHS I resigned to concentrate full time on medico-legal work and, although now retired from police work, I am still involved in a consulting capacity.

From 1974 I was Honorary Secretary of the Association of Police Surgeons of Great Britain, which later dropped the last part of that title as members from all over the world joined the only body to cater for their many and varied needs. I was elected President of the Association in 1994 and still contribute to the field of legal medicine as Immediate Past President.

The public has always had a fascination with forensic medicine. The success of Agatha Christie's legendary detectives in solving their crimes often depended upon the results of laboratory analysis or medical opinion. Today the general public is increasingly better informed on scientific matters and the profile of forensic medicine in popular drama is consequently on the up. Indeed, it often seems today that no television detective can solve any of his or her cases without at least one personal visit to the scene of an autopsy. The *Dangerfield* television series is centred upon the work of a police surgeon who could well have been based in Northamptonshire. The programme first appeared in 1995 and of course proved immensely popular. My own involvement with it as a technical adviser was, and remains, a hugely enjoyable experience. It also made me realise that my work as a police surgeon might well be of wider interest than just to my immediate family circle.

I have been involved in the investigation into nearly all major crimes in Northamptonshire in the past three decades and this has included more than 50 murders.

However, most of my work in the forensic field has been with living patients and victims of crime, and the memories that here make up my story contain a little mystery, a little sex, a little excitement and a little local history – all making for a very enjoyable life. The work has been hard and demanding at times, but it has certainly never been dull!

Hugh de la Haye Davies
September 1998

1

EARLY CASES: ALL FOR A BALE OF HAY

It was a possible murder charge that precipitated my entry into the world of forensic medicine in the 1950s. The case concerned a young Irish labourer who died after being involved in a fight outside the Bat and Wickets, a tavern in Louise Road, Northampton much favoured by the many young Irishmen who were employed in the construction industry, and especially on the new M1 motorway then being built.

He had been struck a blow on the jaw and in falling had hit the back of his head on the pavement, sustaining a fracture which was not at first diagnosed. He died after two or three days in hospital and during this period various bruises sustained in the brawl made their appearance, as well as numerous marks and bruises from the hospital procedures to which he had been subjected for medical investigation and treatment. The pathologist quite correctly for the sake of accuracy and completeness had made a full list in his report, but had stated that in his opinion the injuries were consistent with having been kicked. This was at variance with what the witnesses had observed, in what was described by one as 'a good punch up, which is typical on a Friday night when the Paddies have had a skinful.'

This was my first experience of how medical reports may be interpreted wrongly by lay persons. A loosely

11

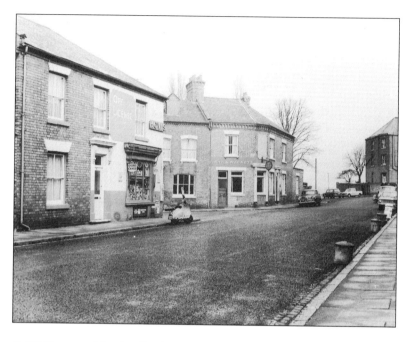

Bailiff Street and Louise Road, Northampton in the 1950s, showing the Bat and Wickets public house. (*Northamptonshire Borough Police*)

worded opinion can lead to disastrous consequences, as in this case when a man involved in the fight was charged with murder. The solicitor asked me if I could arrange for another post mortem, as none of the witnesses had seen anyone use their feet on the deceased.

On studying the report I noted there was a small area of bleeding on the surface of the brain opposite the site where the skull had made contact with the pavement. This was a 'contra coup' haemorrhage which is caused by sudden deceleration of the skull. The significance of this had not been appreciated by the original pathologist but it meant the fracture had been sustained due to the skull hitting the pavement with some force, with the brain travelling on in the same direction inside the now stationary skull. As a consequence small blood vessels going from the inner surface of the skull to the outer surface of the brain on the opposite side had ruptured, leading to the bleeding. This also meant the fractured skull was caused by the fall and not by a kick, grounds sufficient to reduce the charge to the lesser one of manslaughter.

I asked Professor Francis Camps from the world-renowned Department of Forensic Medicine at the London Hospital to carry out the second autopsy. He was famous for his work in the 10 Rillington Place murders and many other cases which had attracted media attention at that time. In the old mortuary at Northampton General Hospital, Camps started work while I took the notes. Looking at us from the other side of the table were the top brass of the Borough CID.

They had not been exactly enthusiastic in welcoming such a distinguished guest to question their original inter-pretation of the post mortem, their looks and body language leaving me in no doubt as to their feelings. I was grateful when Camps boomed out for all in the PM room to hear, 'Dr Davies, you are absolutely correct, this is a classical contra coup haemorrhage.'

Afterwards we repaired to the club just opposite the hospital and a few gin and tonics later I had been persuaded to go on a course he was running for police surgeons to study for the Diploma in Medical Jurispru-dence. I went on the course, passed the exam and started a long association with the London hospital. I became an Honorary Clinical Assistant there, as well as a regular customer at the Blind Beggar pub just across the road from the hospital. This very comfortable and welcoming pub was made famous in the late 1960s by the murder of Jack 'The Hat' McVitie, which eventually led to the conviction of the Kray twins. Many years later when I was a visiting medical officer to HM Prison Gartree I occasionally spoke with Reggie, but refrained from mentioning our mutual place of refreshment. I didn't want to make him homesick.

Forensic medicine has been described as the application of medical knowledge to the administration of the law. The subject is divided into forensic pathology, which deals primarily with the dead, and clinical forensic medicine, which deals with the living.

Police surgeons, or Forensic Medical Examiners as they are now called in many forces, mainly practise forensic medicine, although there is some involvement with pathology as the police have to call a police surgeon to every violent, unexplained or suspicious death. His duty is 'to confirm for police purposes that a body is dead and that there is no prima facie evidence of foul play.' He is the first scientific observer to visit the scene and if he fails to spot the possibility that a crime has been committed, there is every chance that the culprit may well have slipped out of the area or even of the country by the time the alarm is raised.

When I first arrived in Northamptonshire in the 1950s as an assistant in general practice, my senior partner was a prosperous and well-respected GP with a decent sized National Health list as well as a thriving private practice. He was also the County Police Surgeon. Private patients soon became both literally and metaphorically a dying breed, but as one door closes another door opens. By the time I became a full partner, the liberal attitudes of the Sixties and the consequent changes in society had produced a marked increase in police work.

As statistics have proved, half of all work for the 'Old Bill' arises between the hours of midnight and 8 am. Despite this, having found myself a wife I was rather keen to become a permanent fixture in the practice. I therefore at the earliest opportunity declared I had a strong interest in forensic medicine and would be more than happy to take on the police work.

The first case in which my professional opinion was sought involved two young poachers. With their shotguns in the back of their car, they had been in the habit of driving around until they spotted a pheasant. They would shoot it, put it in the boot and drive off quickly to another part of the Northamptonshire countryside where the gamekeepers had not been alerted by the noise of the shot. There were five pheasants in the boot of their car when tragedy struck.

As one of the lads leaned over the back of the passenger seat to pick up his gun, he held the muzzle against his chest, anatomically directly in the region of the heart. The gun, which had a faulty safety catch, went off and he was killed, the shot entering the heart from a direct contact wound. This account was given to the police investigators by his friend, who was known to them but not for anything of a serious nature.

It was important to rule out foul play and the police were not entirely happy with the story. The survivor said that his friend had stood up after the shot and said quite clearly, 'I'm dead!' before he fell.

Examination of the powder-burnt clothing and the wound, with the disruption of the tissues, confirmed that it was a direct contact injury. The angle of entry also fitted with the description given by the witness, but the police were still not convinced that the deceased had been able to so clearly describe his own fate. I was able to reassure them that as the circulation time of blood from heart to brain is something like 23 seconds, there was time for such a sequence of events to occur. This removed any doubts they held as to the veracity of the witness. Although for practical purposes the young man's death could be considered instantaneous, strictly speaking it was not so.

As time went on my increasing involvement in police work naturally had its effect on my family life. Returning home from a police call in the early hours one morning I disturbed my sleeping wife who, half asleep, mumbled as I crawled into bed, 'You had better hurry up and go, Hugh will be back soon.' I still don't know who she was thinking of in her dreams but she claims she was dreaming that one of the children had crept into our bed.

I was on the balance of probabilities prepared to believe her, as all our children quite frequently, on hearing me go out on a night call, got up and moved into my vacated space. On return I often had to content myself with a reduced portion of the bed. As I would be back into a sound sleep within moments of closing my eyes I didn't worry about such matters. In fact, it reassured me that whatever was wrong outside, my own family were safe and sound, for which I was truly thankful.

One such occasion was when I was called to the newly opened M1 where a stolen car had gone under the tail of a heavy goods vehicle parked on the hard shoulder. Two young teenagers had been burned literally to cinders in the resulting conflagration. It was the first of many times I attended incidents on the motorway and I carried out my duties in a professional manner appropriate to the occasion. It was not until I reached my garden gate that the shock and horror of the night registered with me. As I became aware of the smell which I had not noticed at the scene, I was violently sick. An odour of a mixture of burnt flesh and petrol, which had permeated my clothing, was the catalyst in relieving the tension of the previous two hours. Although it has never happened on subsequent occasions, I have been unable to eat roast lamb

16

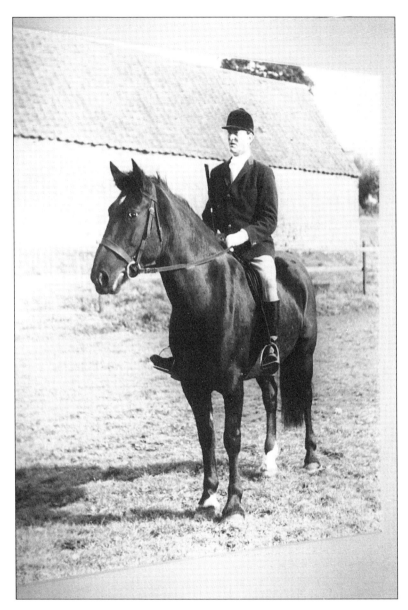

With my favourite horse, Ebony.

ever since unless it is heavily disguised, as the smell reminds me still of that early morning over 30 years ago.

Despite such moments my interest in forensic work increased. Gradually, in a phased withdrawal, first I left the group practice in the town to look after a few hundred or so patients in the country area around my house, then as my medico-legal work increased I eventually had to resign from the NHS.

One week some quarter of a century ago, during a flu epidemic, I had been out every night on police or practice calls. On this particular night I was, at 3.30 am, examining an alleged rape victim. After two hours of meticulous and patient work I was writing my report when I fell asleep at my desk. I was woken by the attending WPC, a charming girl called Linda Spring, bringing a cup of much needed coffee.

'Bad news, Doctor,' she said. 'I'm sorry, but the victim has withdrawn her complaint.' She must have sensed my despair and tiredness because she immediately added, 'Never mind, Doctor, it will buy you a few bales of hay!'

This was in reference to my hobby of keeping horses and the current price of hay, which I had been bemoaning earlier in the evening.

From that day onward the whole of the Northamptonshire Police felt that I was only motivated to provide them with the high quality of service and expertise they expected in order to finance my expensive indulgence in equestrian activities. Many a custody sergeant or CID officer wanting a medical opinion (usually at 3 am) would say, 'We can't get the duty doctor, but this will be worth a few bales of hay for you,' knowing that instant response was almost a certainty.

I make no bones about it, their supposition was usually correct. I could forget the stresses and strains of the job the minute I entered, or even smelled, my stable yard.

Horses and hounds have been my perfect antidote to medicine, both in general practice and forensic work, where one deals with more than one's fair share of human tragedies. On the morning I made the decision to leave the Health Service, my wife said with horror and concern, 'And what are we going to do for money?'

'Have no fear, darling,' I replied. 'The only growth industry in the country today is crime.'

2

ANGEL LANE POLICE STATION AND DRUNKS IN CHARGE

In the 1950s there were still two police forces in the county: the Northampton Borough Police which looked after the County town itself and the Northamptonshire Constabulary which policed the large rural area of the county. This included the smaller towns of Kettering, Corby and Wellingborough in the north and east, with Daventry, Towcester and Brackley in the west and south. All these smaller towns had their own police stations with a resident inspector, and each village had its own police house with a resident constable.

The area around Northampton was policed from Angel Lane, an old Victorian station which was actually in the town centre and thus in the middle of the Borough Police jurisdiction. Most of my work when I started was from Angel Lane, and consisted mainly of examining motorists who were suspected of driving a vehicle when under the influence of drink or drugs.

As most offenders had been brought in to Angel Lane by police car from some distance, many had sobered up by the time they reached the station and completed the various formalities prior to the doctor being called. They had usually come to the notice of the police by the nature of their driving or because they had been in an accident, more often than not something very minor.

20

Usually the initial opinion of the arresting officer would be supported by his colleagues and witnesses at the scene, but successful prosecution required a doctor's opinion that the impairment was due to drink or drugs rather than illness or the effects of the accident, such as concussion.

The doctor doing the police examination was always, in such a small community, in danger of meeting patients or friends. Although I have had to examine medical colleagues on rare occasions, thankfully they have accepted my opinions with good grace – especially as I would take them home afterwards and make arrangements for their vehicles to be delivered home as well! I also followed proper medical etiquette and never charged a fee for services to a colleague.

On one occasion one of them, a very good friend of mine, was asked by one of his own patients if he would attend the station on his, the prisoner's, behalf. Most doctors tactfully decline such private invitations, especially as in many cases they are unlikely to recover their fee, but not Billy, who I suspect was looking forward to getting his own back. I rang him before he set off as I knew he would wait as long as he could to give the chap every chance to sober up, but I wanted reassurance that I was not going to finish up examining him as well, as an encore. He swore he hadn't had a drink that night as he was on duty, and he would arrive one minute before the deadline he had been given by the charge sergeant.

He duly arrived smiling and was shown into the front office, rather than the entrance to the charge room he usually passed through. As he looked at the serious faces of the assembled company he beamed at them and said in his charming Irish brogue, 'Well, gentlemen, it is to be sure a great pleasure to be on the other side for a change.'

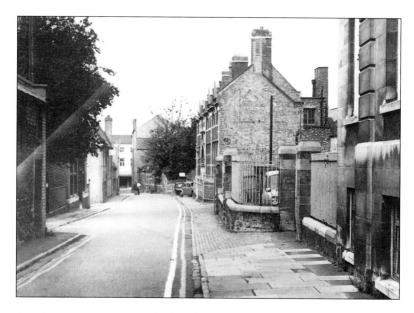

Angel Lane – Northampton's old police station. Centuries ago the town gaol was here too, and executions took place on a gallows in the street. It ceased to be the County Constabulary headquarters in 1963, following a move to Mere Way sub-divisional station. (*Northampton Chronicle & Echo*)

'Don't speak too soon, sir,' responded the charge sergeant. 'You've parked your car on the wrong side of the road and the headlights are full on. If you give me your keys I'll move it for you before one of these keen young lads wakes up and nicks you!'

My first drink-drive case was that of a young farmer who had put his car into the ditch after leaving his local and was blissfully sleeping it off when the police arrived. When I saw him he was being sick in the corner of his cell. An old-fashioned charge sergeant patiently looked on as I attempted to examine the unfortunate lad, who was obviously unable to cooperate with me. It was not possible to carry out the comprehensive medical tests

22

recommended by the British Medical Association handbook on the subject.

After about 20 minutes I turned to the sergeant and said, 'In my opinion he is under the influence of drink to such an extent as to be incapable of having proper control of a motor vehicle.'

The sergeant replied with due courtesy, 'I think you have made a correct diagnosis, Doctor.' I was not sure if he was just being polite or whether he was expressing relief that the new doctor's diagnostic skills were equal to those of the traffic officers.

From Angel Lane the traffic patrol car would travel sometimes as far out as Market Harborough in Leicestershire, a distance of nearly 20 miles, and would often be diverted another 20 miles. I never remember any traffic officers with stress or nervous debility in those balmy days, however, as despite the great amount of mileage covered the pressure of work was nothing like it is today.

My first police casualty came from a traffic patrol who had attended an accident. Three injured men had already been put in the back of the ambulance (which often arrived before the patrol!) but one fatal casualty had been covered with a blanket and left in the ditch where he had been found. Mick was about to check the dead man's identity when the 'corpse' suddenly sat up, groaning.

The victim was recovering from a deep unconscious state, mainly alcohol induced but also contributed to by trauma from the accident. Mick jumped back with such surprise that he caught his ankle on a tree stump and sustained quite a severe Pott's fracture of the ankle. This unfortunately required an operation and I think six months off work, while the original casualties, not having anything to warrant further treatment, were discharged home promptly, including the 'corpse'.

Drink-driving cases formed the largest part of my workload in those days. It was important not only to get the diagnosis correct (which any third year medical student could manage), but also to later stand up in court and present the medical evidence in a fair and unbiased manner. In many cases there were doubts and quite rightly the defence lawyer would probe deeply into these, as he was the voice for his client. The doctor had to make sure that the court was made aware of alternative explanations, but equally to stand firm where he was certain beyond a reasonable doubt.

The mythology surrounding the examination includes the belief that the accused had to walk a white line. This is not strictly true, as although most of the older charge rooms have a white line marked on the floor, it is historical decoration rather than there to serve any useful purpose. Asking the person to walk across the room was included in the general examination as the doctor could assess their gait as part of deciding whether coordination had been affected. The tests for this could not be too difficult as defence counsel would soon make much of the fact that the tests were therefore unfair, or even biased to get a conviction. 'After all, Doctor, it is the police who pay you,' might be suggested or implied.

It is quite difficult for some people even when stone cold sober to walk exactly a straight line, especially if they are nervous. Asking them to just walk to the other side of the room, turn around and then walk back would soon demonstrate a staggering or unstable gait. This then had to be differentiated from the person's normal gait which might be affected by a natural disease such as arthritis. The most amusing and unsuccessful explanation put forward by one defence solicitor to explain his client's wide unsteady gait was that his client suffered from prolapsed piles and was on the hospital waiting list

24

for them to be attended to. My offer to examine the prisoner was, in view of collateral evidence, declined by their Worships when they found the accused guilty.

One test that was helpful in persons who could read and write was to ask them to copy out something such as a few sentences from the Highway Code or a local newspaper. It was quite often said in a person's defence that this test was unfair because the client was not well educated and was also nervous. On one occasion when an educated man had obviously written in a drunken scrawl, I wrote a note on the exhibit to the effect that it was written in my presence by the man and the times he had started and finished. The chairman of the Quarter Sessions was Sir Reginald Manningham-Buller MP (known to his parliamentary colleagues as Bullying Manner). He was a former Attorney General. He looked at this paper, exhibit number one, before handing it to the jury and said, 'Can you please show the court, Doctor, which is your writing and which is the defendant's?' He was not, as I first thought, making a judicial jest at my expense. It was in fact necessary under the rules of evidence that the exhibit be properly proved.

On another occasion when I was appearing for the defence, the accused complained that he had found difficulty in first reading the piece and then writing it because he had not had his glasses with him at the time. The certifying police surgeon should have conceded that this was a possible explanation for the slightly irregular and illegible calligraphy but stubbornly refused to do so, despite gentlemanly suggestions by our counsel. On my suggestion he was handed a copy of the Highway Code and asked first to read from it with his glasses on, then to remove his glasses and repeat the exercise. The whole court observed the way he had to move the script further away from his eyes until it was at arm's length before he could read it. He conceded our point before we had to ask him to write anything.

It was common knowledge that many guilty persons got off because we had to concede that clinical examination on its own without the benefit of biochemical tests was neither sufficiently reliable nor sensitive enough to confirm impairment through drunk or drugs. It was this 'sporting element' of British justice which resulted in so many acquittals, and led to the introduction of the breathalyser under the Road Traffic Act of 1967. Everything is so relatively simple these days! As long as you are competent enough to find a vein that does not collapse and you can get a sample of blood which is then analysed, the result is clear cut one way or the other.

In the old days there would be at least one solicitor in each town who specialised in drink-driving cases, and who saw it as his public duty to educate both young and old police surgeons. Out of court he would probably be a member of the same golf club or masonic lodge as the doctor, and in many cases possibly the accused as well. However, once in court he had only one objective and that was to get his client off at all costs. His reputation was at stake and with the reporters from the local press hanging on his every word, his delivery was timed to the speed of the pencils of the press bench.

A good opening gambit would be to produce the 'Blue Book'. This was the BMA's official publication entitled *The Recognition of Intoxication.* It was the report of a BMA special committee, 39 pages long in a blue cover and priced one shilling and sixpence. I fortunately bought one as soon as I took up police work, but it was surprising how many doctors didn't. They soon found out to their cost that every defence lawyer had one and used it as tablets of stone.

I well remember the late Harry Skinner QC (eventually

he became a High Court judge) arguing a point with me and holding the Blue Book in the air, waving it at the jury and saying, 'It says so in your book, Doctor.' Then to emphasise the point, he waved his arms in a dramatic gesture and fixed the jury with his beady eye. '*Your* book, Doctor, not mine.'

I think I muttered something about 'circumstances altered cases and there were exceptions to the book'. Quick as a flash he was on his feet and turning to the jury said, 'So this doctor considers he can give an alternative view than that held by a special committee of the BMA!' He then sat down quickly after saying, 'No more questions, Your Honour.' He had made his point and not surprisingly his client was acquitted.

The Blue Book was also used against me early on in my career in the case of a local businessman who had had his own doctor present during the examination. Needless to say, this was his private not his NHS doctor. I took a lot of trouble and as the BMA recommended 40 tests that could form part of the full and thorough examination I performed them all – mainly for the benefit of the private doctor, who I suspect realised very early on that his patient was somewhat tired and emotional, to say the least.

At the court hearing some three months later the doctor did not appear, but with horror I recognised the same solicitor who had in the case of the young farmer mentioned earlier, well criticised me for saying his client was drunk when I had only carried out three of those tests, despite my protestations that it was impossible to do any more. This time I felt I was on stronger ground, but not surprisingly the defence cross-examination started with, 'Really Doctor, you must admit this was a very borderline case, wasn't it? You had to carry out all 40 tests before you could say my client was drunk!'

27

Despite the theatrical pauses and the emphasis on the words 'borderline' and 'forty', their Worships found his client guilty. The case did not go to appeal.

In 1959 Angel Lane was replaced by a more modern station to cater for the needs of both the local area and those of the newly opened M1, the first part of the country's motorway network. The new station was built at Mere Way on the southern edge of the town and only three miles on a fast dual carriageway from the M1's junction 15. It is still the home of the Traffic Division, with alongside it both an ambulance station and a fire station. County Police headquarters and my new office were situated in Wootton Hall Park adjoining this complex, so that if I heard the sirens of all three services I knew that in a short time I could expect a call myself. In 1965 the two police forces in the county combined and my partner and I also took on responsibility for the more heavily populated area of the Borough.

Angel Lane had been Victorian in structure but a cosy station to work from. Although it had no such thing as a doctor's room, the charge room was perfectly adequate for most examinations. In the event that you needed to examine someone lying down, recourse was made to the very wide and long seat that ran alongside the wall of the billiards room. With a rolled up policeman's cape for a pillow and a blanket from the cell stores, it made a very functional substitute for a surgery couch (which we were able to obtain after special pleading at the new station at Mere Way). A room was also set aside specially for the doctor's use, but it had to be shared with the fingerprint department.

These days it is usual practise for police stations to have properly equipped medical rooms, but then it was the exception rather than the rule. At night if you needed a chaperone for a female patient, the inspector's wife, who lived with her husband and family on the top floor of the station, would get up and oblige if the station WPC was off duty.

It was then also normal practice in the County forces for the wife to live 'over the job', where she was expected to answer the telephone and perform other duties to assist her husband. Here there is a similarity with doctors' wives, but at least I did not have to have the permission of my senior partner before I took my spouse to the altar, whereas police officers had to have the Chief Constable's approval. This was usually given after a full enquiry into the suitability of the prospective bride as a wife in his force. In these days of equal opportunities and political correctness the policemen do not have the benefit of such wise counsel, and I wonder if some will say they have learned to regret it!

3

DANGERS OF
THE OLDEST PROFESSION

Northampton, like all large towns, has always had a number of ladies engaged in the oldest profession, prostitution. During the Second World War the influx of American servicemen into the area and the surrounding counties was a factor in making the town a mecca for prostitutes from all parts of the Midlands.

In those days there was a deeply religious Chief Constable who, I have been told by some of his officers, acknowledged the problem but was of the opinion that no amount of policing would stop it. He did not make it a priority in either time or money, and was heard to express the view that it was easier to contain the problem than to try and eradicate it. A certain area of the town, now redeveloped, became the centre of their activities and here there was little or no police harassment. His view was shared by many, who also believed that having the vice contained in one area would make it safer elsewhere, especially for women and children.

Today many things have changed in the way the 'game' is played. Many of the girls are now deeply involved with the drugs scene, and their activities are also a part of protection rackets controlled by pimps and ponces. It is a dangerous occupation, more so now than it has ever been.

I first met Barbara when she was aged 28. She had

been on the game for about ten years, but had not lost her good looks or pleasant personality. She was known to the police, but only had a few minor convictions. She had been brought in as a victim of alleged attempted murder.

Barbara's story began when, after placing his money on her bedside table, a punter had taken some time to proceed with what he had paid for. She remarked to him that time was money to her and would he get on with it.

She remembered: 'He put his hands around my neck and gripped tight. I went hazy and saw black, my head was throbbing, my Adam's apple was being pressed back. I punched him and pulled his hair, then I must have passed out as the next thing I remember is being sick and blood was coming out of my mouth or nose, not much blood but it was on the cushion.'

Her client had not only departed in haste, leaving her for dead, but had also taken his money back.

The details she recounted suggested that this was indeed attempted strangulation and not merely accidental or a session of vigorous loveplay, as the lawyers often suggest in such cases. This was a deliberate, forceful attempt to kill.

I remember Barbara well because she was my first such case where the physical findings clearly corroborated the story of the victim. Her face was covered with petechial haemorrhages looking rather like a measles rash, and she had extensive sub-conjunctival haemorrhages in both eyes, all consistent with asphyxia due to obstructed venous return from the neck. There were numerous bruises and scratches around both sides of her neck, some from the fingernails and thumbs of the assailant while others were inflicted by Barbara in her efforts to free herself. The man was never caught.

I next saw Barbara nearly four years later when she

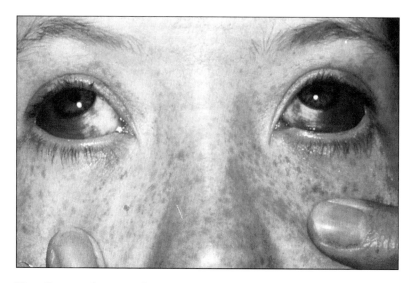

The effect on the eyes of attempted strangulation. When the veins from the head are compressed in the neck, pressure builds up in the minute capillaries under the facial skin and in the front of the eyes. These eventually burst producing small fine haemorrhages under the skin (petechial haemorrhages) and subconjunctival haemorrhages in the eyes. These may be obvious as in this case but can be very slight and only observed when the lower eyelids are retracted. This picture taken by the late Dr Stanley Burges appears in an Association of Police Surgeons' publication entitled *Rape*.

was lying unconscious in the local hospital's casualty department. Detective Constable Vickers had a grim look on his face as he met me there at one-thirty in the morning.

'Sorry to get you out so early, Doc,' he explained, 'but they found her in an alleyway off the Wellingborough Road. The hospital doctor thinks she might die.'

On examination her body was found to be covered with massive bruising and there were also marks around her neck. She was deeply unconscious. From a reconstruction of her multiple injuries I formed the opinion that

32

she had been battered around the head and face with a blunt instrument.

On the back and front of her trunk there were criss-cross lacerations consistent with her having been dragged unclothed across broken glass. Bruises on her neck were classic strangulation marks. Injuries to her head could have been caused by it being struck with great force against a wall or floor. She was a very slightly built girl and none of her injuries could have been the result of her falling down when drunk, as was suggested by the defence at the subsequent trial.

Fortunately, she recovered consciousness after a week and at the trial her assailant was found guilty of grievous bodily harm and sentenced to three years. Barbara was still under hospital care and I don't know if she ever recovered completely, as at the trial she was showing signs of residual brain damage.

Barbara was lucky to survive. These women who practise the oldest profession live dangerously and often die violently. They have been providing media copy since the days of Jack the Ripper and will probably continue to do so. One such case I was involved with in 1971 was dubbed by the press 'The Hot Pants Murder at the Welcome Inn'.

The landlord of the Welcome public house was a married man of good character who lived with his wife and five children above the bar. He was known as a mild, hard-working man who despite some of his clientele, which in those days included some of the town's prostitutes and their customers, ran a well ordered house which had given no concern to the police or the licensing authority.

On the night of Wednesday, 17th November 1971 a local lad who was a regular customer and also a singer at the pub mentioned that he was looking for a car. The

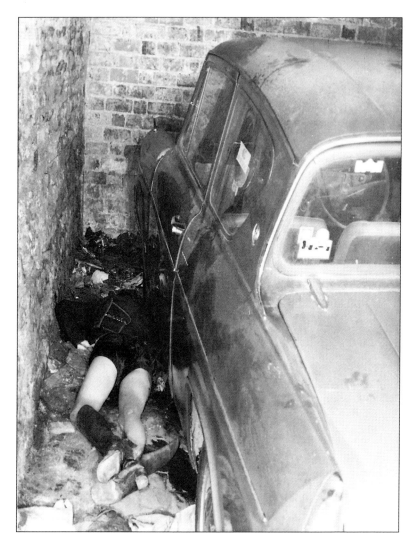

The body of Heather Campbell was found in a garage at the Welcome Inn in 1971 – a case dubbed 'The Hot Pants Murder' by the press. The right knee-length boot where she was alleged to keep her money was found to be zipped open when she was discovered. (*Northamptonshire and County Constabulary*)

landlord said he had one he wanted to sell and took him round to the back of the pub.

The garage was dark and as the lad, Lawrence McCann, felt his way round the car his foot kicked something soft. It was the body of Heather Campbell, a well known local prostitute. She was dressed in a leather-type short jacket, short velvet pants (known then as hot pants) and a pair of knee-length boots. She was lying in a pool of blood between the car and the wall. Her right boot was unzipped but her tights were still firmly in place, while it was later discovered her right hand grasped a packet of contraceptives.

The police were called and the first officer on the scene, Constable John Ruff, immediately sealed off the garage. The investigating team then arrived, at first under the command of Detective Superintendent Arthur Crawley and his assistant Detective Chief Inspector Geoff Carter. They took over the lounge bar as the site control and divided the detectives into teams to start preliminary questioning of customers in the adjoining bar and surrounding area.

I came on the scene together with Detective Inspector Norman Edmunds, who was in charge of the crime team of fingerprint experts and photographers. Detective Superintendent Brian Scarth arrived from Force head-quarters and, just before closing time, bought us all a drink.

I was impressed at the time not by the fact that the most senior officer, who had come to take overall command, had bought us a drink, but by the reaction of the landlord. As he handed Brian the change he said, 'I've no need to remind you gentlemen that it will soon be drinking-up time and I would be obliged if you would make sure your glasses are empty as I've got some stock-taking to attend to before I go to bed.'

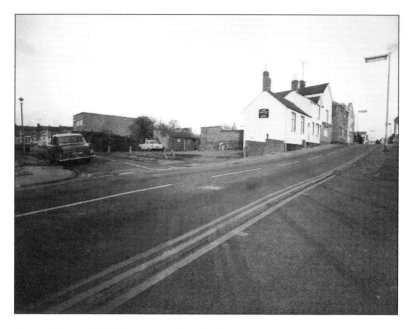

General view of the Welcome Inn from Grafton Street.

I thought his response odd to say the least. After all, it's not every day you discover a corpse in your garage and have a murder enquiry based in your pub lounge!

Meanwhile, an interesting snippet had been picked up by a detective when talking to the local prostitutes. One of them was quite sure that not only did the dead girl visit the pub quite often, but also that the landlord used her services. He had claimed that he did not know the dead girl – though this is often a natural first reaction when family men are questioned in relation to any matters involving prostitutes. It would obviously need to be checked out.

We waited in the lounge for the arrival of Peter Andrews, our Home Office pathologist, and also Norman

Lee, the forensic scientist who had to come from the laboratory at Nottingham. On the way his car broke down on the motorway and he arrived in style, towed by a brand new Traffic Department Range Rover! In the meantime, an incident room had been set up at Campbell Square station just up the road and the team had started analysing the first of several hundred statements to be taken from pub customers, prostitutes and their clients (many under a pledge of secrecy), as well as others who had known Heather.

After a fortnight a picture had been built up of a girl whose real name was Naomi Phinn, last seen alive on the evening of 16th November. She was separated from her husband, who was left behind in Glasgow when she came south to live in nearby Rugby, and was known as a tough cookie who regularly worked in the town.

Peter Andrews confirmed that she had been struck at least five times with a blunt object about the head and face. Death was due to shock and haemorrhage following severe, penetrating head wounds. In Peter's view, if she had been found earlier she might have been saved. The instrument was shown to be a hammer, the head of which was found at the scene. It was also learned that she used to put her earnings inside her right knee-length boot, which was found unzipped.

Forensic evidence soon proved the link between the landlord and Heather Campbell, including a banknote found at his home stained with blood of the same group as the victim. He was arrested and charged with murder.

At the trial he admitted he had been a client of Heather's, but the defence case was based on his claim that she was blackmailing him by threatening to tell his wife. He had paid her increasing amounts of money, leading to financial problems with his business. That evening he had taken her to the garage on the pretext of having sex with her, but also to discuss her demands. On the way out he saw the hammer under the bar and put it in his pocket. When she asked again for money, he said, he temporarily lost control of himself and hit her with the hammer.

He was found not guilty of murder but guilty of manslaughter, for which he was sentenced to eight years. Mr Justice Ackner described the verdict as merciful, 'for as bad a case of manslaughter as one ever saw'.

I have mentioned some of the officers involved in the Hot Pants Murder case as this was the first time I had worked as a team with Dr Peter Andrews and forensic scientist Norman Lee. Little did any of us realise as we sat in the lounge of the Welcome Inn that cold November night with the body of Heather Campbell only a few yards away, that we would be working together over the next ten years on more than 50 murders. Only two of those cases remain unsolved but we have still not closed the files. Although I was the last to retire of that little band, who knows but that someday our successors may yet be in a position to do so.

One thing is certain – those who follow the oldest profession lead dangerous lives. I have often been asked why they do it. Apart from those in recent years who need to finance their drug habit, there are those who are in the grip of so-called boyfriends or partners to whom they have to give most of their earnings. Then there are those, and many of them, who do it for the sake of their family – who need to pay a large household bill or raise the money to send a child on a school trip. More so today than when I first started in practice, there seem to be single mothers and those whose husbands are out of work, so that they become ensnared in the poverty trap. Such a woman was the subject of my last case of

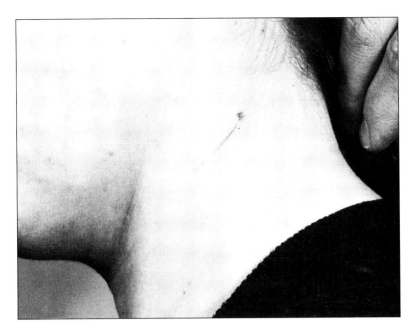

Scratch marks on the neck corroborate a woman's claim that a man had held a knife to her neck and were sustained when she turned to look at him as she grasped the knife. The cut on the inside of the middle part of the thumb is a typical defence injury.

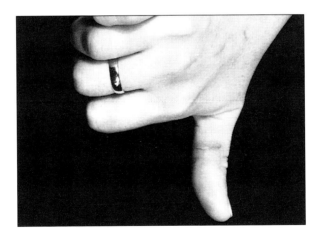

attempted murder, examined in the final month of my service with the police.

Tracy worked as a masseuse, offering the usual services at clients' houses. After a response to one of her advertisements in a local paper, she visited a house where the client appeared to remain unsatisfied – due to his own inadequacy rather than failure on Tracy's part, it has to be said.

Being a professional, Tracy offered him his money back if he felt the service was not up to the standard he expected. His response, she told the jury at his trial, was to say, 'Now you slut, the time has come for you to die.' He then put his hands around her neck and squeezed. She remembered fighting with him to try and release the pressure but with little success until they fell struggling off the bed. At this stage she was able to break free and ran naked into the street. A neighbour who had heard her screams had dialled 999 and was waiting with her as the police car arrived.

I examined her the next day with a WPC in attendance, who had prepared Tracy with a full explanation as to the reason for her seeing a doctor, especially the hope that we might find some evidence to corroborate her allegations. As a result Tracy was most helpful, particularly after being told she was in command of the situation and that nothing would be done to her during the examination without her consent.

This has been a routine I have followed with all my patients, especially the children though it must be remembered that adults are also nervous when they see a doctor in such circumstances. The most important consideration is a sensitivity to the needs of the victim. While the gender of the doctor is not as important as their competence to collect the evidence and present it in an unbiased way to the court, if necessary being able to withstand cross-examination, if a female victim is uncomfortable with being examined by a male doctor then it is now the policy in most police forces to try and find a properly trained female doctor instead. The same applies to male victims or prisoners. It is sometimes still not realised that a sympathetic and understanding attitude on the part of the doctor and police officers who deal with the victim can often be the first stage in his or her therapy. This has been recognised by the Northamptonshire Police for many years and both myself and the local Rape Crisis Centre have regular input into the police training programme.

My findings in Tracy's case were not as outstanding as I have described for Barbara earlier, but were certainly enough to corroborate her allegations and to demonstrate that the force used against her was not accidental but with intent. A guilty verdict was returned and her attacker was sentenced to seven years.

I have had to examine many women over the years who have been victims of violence, and I have also been called in when it has been necessary to declare them fit to be detained and interviewed if picked up for crimes not related to prostitution, such as shoplifting to provide for their drug habits. As a result I became quite well known to them.

Peter Green, a prominent forensic medical examiner with the Metropolitan Police, works mainly at busy Brixton police station. He was called one night to confirm that a lady from Northampton who had been arrested on a warrant was fit to be taken back there under escort. He reassured her that on her return she would get the very best of medical care as the police surgeon was a friend of his.

'He's a friend of mine too,' the lady replied. 'We all know Hugh. He sees us more than our own doctors and you don't have to wait three days for an appointment!'

Quite true, as they attended with regular frequency, although not usually in a voluntary capacity. Just like some patients in general practice they would soon say, 'And while I'm here, doctor...', leading into a private consultation at the Chief Constable's expense.

It occasionally takes some explaining when, walking through town, I am greeted with a friendly smile and a cheery word or two. And it can sometimes be embarrassing if I am in conversation with some young lady and cannot remember where we have met before. My mental gymnastics as I try to place the face are a source of great amusement to my wife!

4

BLUES AND TWOS EMERGENCIES

Over the years I have worked for many hours and on many different occasions with the emergency services, and no matter how many times one sees the flashing blue lights and hears the two-tone sirens, it always gives a rush of adrenaline into the system.

The need to call a doctor out to serious road traffic accidents has almost disappeared as a result of the increase in numbers of highly trained paramedics and improved response times to emergency call-outs. But this is only in recent times. Motorway accidents and accident investigation were unfortunately specialties in which the Northamptonshire Police gained plenty of practical experience after the opening of the M1 in 1959 and during the first 25 years of the M1 motorway I would usually be called out about once a month.

When John Mayes retired as Chief Inspector (Traffic), he had worked his way up from service as a motorway patrolman in the early days of the motorway. He retired as one of the leading traffic experts in the country, with a real understanding of engineering and traffic problems. A dedicated enthusiast for his chosen specialty, he lectured to police forces all over the country and overseas.

I first met John in the early days of the M1 when there were no central crash barriers. Traffic was very light

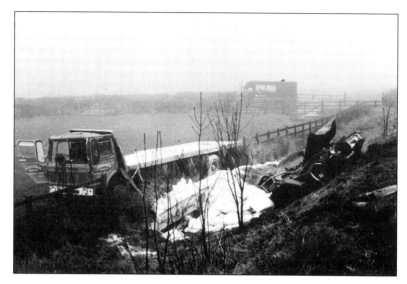

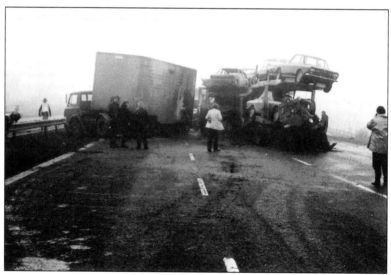

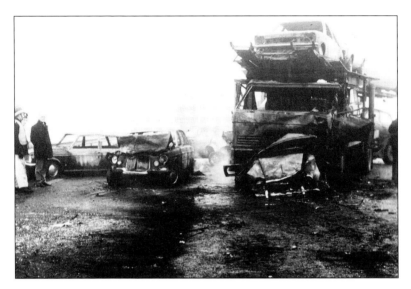

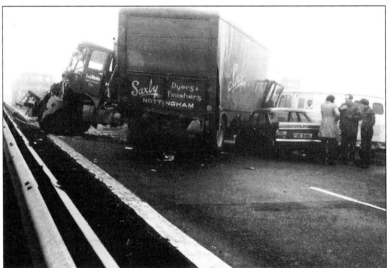

The dreadful consequences of the multiple crash at the Crick interchange on the M1 in 1974.

compared with today's moving traffic jams. If there was an accident on the northbound carriageway and I had driven down the southbound, then it was perfectly possible to park my car, cross on foot at a brisk pace to the central reservation, pause for a moment and then cross over to the opposite side. A traffic officer would meet me to guide me across and carry my bag. Those balmy days have long since gone.

Never to be forgotten by either John or I was the day in March 1974 when 204 vehicles collided in the vicinity of junction 18, the Crick interchange. I believe it is still the largest number of vehicles to have been involved in such a pile-up. Although there were six fatalities and 28 people injured, the hospitals at Rugby and Northampton were fortunately able to cope without much disruption to their normal routine. For the police, together with the fire and rescue services, the event was a major disaster as 14 miles of carriageway were covered with the wrecked cars, many of which caught fire.

The day was very foggy with visibility down to 25 yards but police vehicles using their blue lights on their way to the scene were being overtaken by other drivers travelling too fast and too close, unaware of what lay awaiting them and ignoring police efforts to slow them down.

On arrival at the Crick interchange I transferred to John's vehicle. We came across one large car transporter carrying about eight cars, all on fire, and embedded underneath was a small car, also on fire and in which the driver and passenger had perished. The area round the transporter was the centre of a fireball involving several crashed vehicles. Just within a few feet of the rear wheels of the transporter a lorry had jack-knifed. It was later found to be carrying 60 drums of acetone, which is highly inflammable and in such circumstances, highly explosive.

The loss of life would have been much greater and the damage more widespread if the flames from the transporter had travelled just a few more feet and ignited that lethal cargo, which was being carried without any of the usual Hazchem warning signs.

We spent some considerable time trying to release a driver trapped by his legs in a large Volvo lorry. As the firemen toiled with their cutting device to disengage his legs, which both had compound fractures, we learned by experience how strong is the steel they put in Volvos!

I had sent for the hospital team with a view to amputation as the only way to get the chap out. He was conscious throughout but I administered a mixture of gas and air called Entonox, which I used on many occasions to provide considerable relief to people trapped in such circumstances. Doctors are not enthusiastic about administering morphine or similar drugs at a time like this, and Entonox is a much safer way of putting the patient temporarily into a state of pain-free oblivion. They soon regain consciousness when the mask is removed or, if they hold the mask themselves, can take deep breaths when they feel pain and then the mask will drop from their face when they fall asleep.

In between manipulations by the rescuers my patient became quite conversational and asked many questions about the Entonox, which fortunately in the circumstances had made him quite euphoric. During the conversation I mentioned that I normally used it for women in labour, which brought the immediate response, in the colourful language appropriate to the situation, that if he had a baby he would certainly be a medical miracle.

Soon after that he was released without the necessity for amputation. A couple of days later when he was well on the mend John and I visited him in hospital and he reminded us of this conversation. John commented that we had accomplished the impossible, but miracles take a little longer!

Of the many RTAs – road traffic accidents – that I attended, both on and off the motorway, one that I will never forget involved a personal friend of mine. Maurice Fitch owes his life to the fact that I had dined well that night, enjoying in the process the best part of a bottle of very fine claret.

It was a Saturday and I had had a good day's hunting on my trusty Irish mare Ebony. I was off duty and we had just reached the sweet course when the telephone rang. It was the incident room from Campbell Square. After a rather difficult murder enquiry they had just detained their prime suspect and they required an urgent forensic examination. I felt it prudent to ask for transport to the station, especially as it was a cold and frosty night with patchy fog in places.

On the way in I drew the attention of the officers to a patch of water on the road. A roadside horse trough had overflowed and a drain become blocked with fallen leaves, so the water formed a large pool over the surface of the road. As it was downhill the pool extended to the next functioning drain some 20 yards away.

Four hours later, being transported home in a traffic car, I mentioned the possibility of ice on the road to the driver when we were about a mile from the hazard. As we approached we saw the rear lights of the car in front suddenly veer to the offside as it came up to the blind bend ahead. The police driver slowed down and approached the bend in low gear, almost at a crawl. We could feel our wheels slipping even though the driver was not braking or accelerating.

The car in front had come to rest on the bank on the nearside of the road, having demolished about ten yards of the post and rail fence. Maurice Fitch was the only occupant, lying in the driver's seat semi-conscious. His head was slumped forward on his chest but he was able to say, 'Hello, Doc' as I took his pulse through the driver's window, which somehow one of the policemen had managed to force open. The other called in for assistance to protect the scene and save other drivers coming to grief, and for the fire brigade and ambulance.

Fortunately at that early hour in the morning there was practically no traffic, so the emergency services were on the scene within about 10 to 15 minutes, their blue flashing lights giving timely warning to approaching vehicles. These included a coachload of returning party-goers who managed to stop before hitting the ice.

As for Maurice, he was in reasonably good shape and had realised that we could not open the door because of bits of demolished fence getting in the way. He even explained that he had a chainsaw in the boot if anyone could use it, but a second or two later I firmly declined his offer as I made a discovery that really pushed the adrenaline into my system.

I had cut his safety belt and he had lifted his head spontaneously in turning to speak to us. Warning him to lie still I followed the routine of running my hands down his body, as I had taught so many times at first aid classes. I was looking for the sticky dampness which might indicate bleeding and feeling for any deformity to indicate a possible fracture. I started with the head, then the neck, down to the chest, back and front. Next the collar bones and down the arms. I decided that both elbows and forearms were perfectly normal and I had managed to free them from his sides when I felt what seemed to be another elbow on the left side of his abdomen. As I ran my hands across to the opposite side of his body I felt coarse fencing wood and by the light of the police torch I saw with horror that one of the rails had gone through the door and perforated Maurice's abdomen. The lump I had thought was an elbow was the end of the rail, protruding outwards under his skin.

The fire brigade arrived fairly quickly and it was decided I would hold the piece of wood close to the entry wound to prevent any further movement. A pair of strong firemen's hands gave support next to mine and, as it happened, within a couple of inches of the mechanical saw.

I cannot remember much about the next few minutes, but I do remember in the back of the ambulance looking at the protruding rail and asking the paramedic to hold it tightly as my hands had suddenly lost all their strength. He carefully, and without moving the wood, relieved my grip and held it steady as a rock as the ambulance drove at speed (but with perfect steadiness) to the hospital. The surgeon removed a piece of wooden fencing post 15 inches long and three inches wide, which he said in his report was gradually eased out of the abdominal cavity. There were many other serious internal injuries but these were methodically and slowly repaired all through the night and Maurice was put into the intensive care ward just as the dawn was breaking.

Being as strong as an ox prior to the accident, despite the severity of his injuries Maurice returned to work within the year, building up his tree surgeon business and doing general farm work. A year later the surgeon wrote in a report: 'Apart from some mild discomfort over the site of the scar, he has no abdominal symptoms. He finds that sheep shearing is difficult due to weakness of his left thigh as he is unable to hold the sheep easily.'

This may explain why as you drive around some areas of Northamptonshire, in certain fields the sheep appear to have unusual hairstyles.

The adrenaline that surges into the system as you get

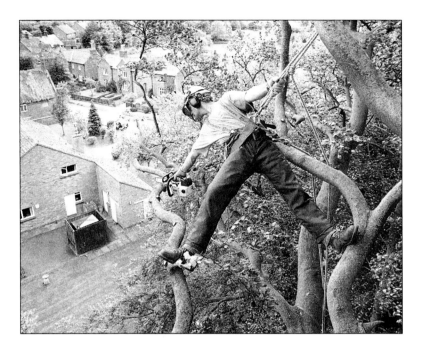

Maurice Fitch, now in very good health and in action over the village of Great Brington on the edge of the Althorp estate. (*Bob Thomas*)

to grips with an emergency situation has certain effects which vary between individuals. In my case, I find that it brings out the best in my training and experience, as whatever the circumstances my mind concentrates on the job in hand to the exclusion of all distractions. So much so, that I often cannot remember exactly what I did and when, although from the evidence of others I evidently did the right thing at the right time.

This is a phenomenon that is well recognised by those who have to debrief emergency personnel after incidents, and one particular case illustrates how memory can play some strange tricks. It was an occasion when I was

51

working with the fire and rescue tender from Long Buckby. This is a part-time brigade made up from firemen who, rather like lifeboatmen, have regular jobs and answer calls in response to a bleep they carry with them at all hours of the day and night (although at the time I am talking about they were still summoned by siren). Until a few years ago the Long Buckby brigade had responded to more motorway calls than any other brigade in the country. However, with reorganisation the rescue tender has been moved to Daventry, a full-time station which has taken over prime response to calls from the motorway.

On this particular day they were working with Blue Watch from Northampton to release a lady trapped in a serious RTA. It was difficult and I slipped my hand around her feet and ankles to assess the problem. A fireman held back a piece of metal superstructure with one hand while with the other he held a torch to provide illumination for the dark and deep hole I was working in. Eventually she was released, though unfortunately she had to have her lower leg amputated later in hospital.

Two days later I met one of my oldest friends, Colin Stephenson. At the time Colin was on Blue Watch and more than once we had been at accident scenes together. I remarked when I saw him that I had attended the incident above, and asked why he had not been there.

'Don't you remember?' he replied. 'I was holding the light for you.'

I had been so engrossed in what I was doing at the time that it had not registered, or if it had then I had completely forgotten about it. This 'adrenaline effect' may well affect the reliability of statements of witnesses to any traumatic event – a fact well known to lawyers. It is a valid reason for conducting in court what may appear to the witness a rather penetrating and unnecessary cross-examination.

My association with the emergency services has involved me in other dramatic situations. In the early evening of Saturday, 17th december 1977, when again I was off duty, the telephone rang. It was the Corby police. They could not find a doctor anywhere in their part of the county so had turned to me for help. I agreed to attend but told them it would be necessary to send a car for me. I was just finishing my high tea when the car came up the drive. At the station a party of wedding guests were finishing their celebrations in the waiting area, while their driver was inside awaiting my attention.

I had completed the routine task of obtaining a blood sample from him and we were on our way back home, when the control room came on the wireless and asked if we could proceed to Kingsthorpe Hollow in North-ampton. The firearms section had been deployed and it was decided the presence of a doctor would be prudent, as is often the case when this section is called out.

When we arrived the area had been cordoned off and armed police had surrounded a gun shop known as the Sportsman's Lodge. An ambulance and two fire engines were in attendance. This was at the time of the Fire Brigade's industrial dispute and the fire engines were manned by the Army and known from their colour as 'Green Goddesses'. The reason for the alert was that a young man had been caught breaking in to the gun shop and was refusing to come out.

Detective Chief Inspector Peter Sharpe, whose family had for many years been patients in my town practice, was at the scene. He greeted me with the up-to-date report on the situation. One of the advantages of having so many police officers and their families on my list was that at times such as this instant rapport was achieved.

My job in such situations was to stay quietly in the background, the Incident Officer knowing I was there, and to be prepared to do whatever he asked of me. Chief Superintendent George Swain, who was in command that night, asked me to join Peter, who was in the post office next door to the gun shop and trying to communicate with the young intruder. Peter, trained to negotiate in such incidents, was one of the few who were available in each police force especially for siege situations. The sieges of the Iranian Embassy, Balcombe Street, and the Spaghetti House had given the Metropolitan Police an opportunity to learn lessons which were, in turn, passed on to police forces all over the country.

As Peter talked through a loudhailer, the youth's behaviour became erratic and more excitable. His father had been brought to the scene and in a brief few minutes I was able to discover a few details of his son's personal and medical history. Then shots began ringing out from the darkened gunshop.

I had made the decision that the youth appeared to be a grossly disturbed psychopath whose unpredictable behaviour could easily endanger both himself and others. After listening to more staccato shouting, both Peter and I decided that no amount of talking was going to lead to a peaceful outcome. In the London sieges there had been dissident groups who made rational demands capable of being carried out, but our character made none. His behaviour was irrational, unpredictable and aggressive.

Just then one of the armed policemen fired a CS gas canister into the shop in a bid to force the youth out. The round exploded and a flash ignited loose cartridge powder which had been scattered during the youth's rampage around the inside of the shop. A blaze very soon flared up. Unfortunately, the two Green Goddesses had been diverted to a fish and chip shop fire and it was not long before it became obvious that the gun shop premises were beyond saving. The best that could be

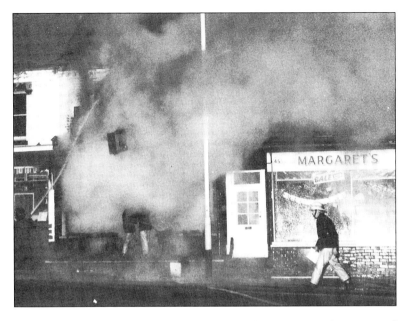

Smoke and exploding ammunition hampered firefighters attempting to control the fire.

hoped for was that when the firefighters returned the fire could be contained and prevented from spreading to neighbouring premises.

In the meantime the firing had abruptly stopped as the youth escaped upstairs in the blazing and smoke-filled building. Explosions from ignited cartridges and boxes of powder rent the air as, through the shop window, the staircase was seen to be well and truly ablaze. Peter and I, sheltering by the dividing wall in the neighbouring post office, decided to leave our position and after seeing the inhabitants safely evacuated, were in time to see the fire tenders return. This time they had with them a rescue tender manned by Royal Navy damage control men who had also been seconded to the brigade during the indus-

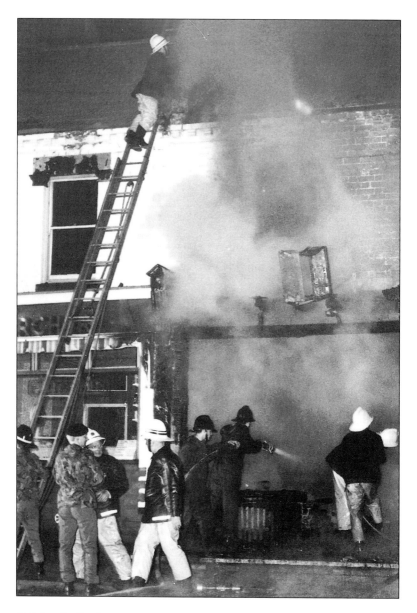

Fighting the fire that resulted from the Kingsthorpe Siege in 1977.

trial action. Engines from two part-time stations outside the town also arrived, and the next door premises were saved.

As black, acrid smoke billowed from the back of the house the youth could be seen trying to get out, but his escape was prevented by a burglar-proof iron grille. When the Navy men managed to remove the bars over the back window, one of their number found the unconscious youth lying on the floor of the room with flames already licking the floorboards. Inspector Tony Wright of the police support group had also gone into the room and he had to be helped out overcome by the smoke.

We were transported to hospital in the same ambulance and Tony recovered enough to be able to help us to restrain the prisoner. As we entered the casualty department he became quite violent. He was later sentenced to life imprisonment.

There was a sequel to this when the insurers of the gunshop took out a writ against the Chief Constable for alleged negligence, as the CS cartridge had been fired while the Green Goddesses were not in attendance. I was called as a witness to explain that the state of mind of the youth at the time the cartridge was fired was such that he had been likely to have broken out of the shop carrying a loaded gun, at considerable risk to those in the vicinity. Unfortunately, despite the highly professional and gallant way the police had coped with the situation that night, in the cold light of day in the High Court some several years later they were found negligent. All because they had not waited for the Green Goddesses to return from the fish and chip shop fire before they fired the errant cartridge.

A moment of light relief occurred during the proceedings when one devoted dog handler described how his faithful hound had gallantly entered the burning premises to search out the youth but had had to exit rapidly because of the intense heat. The next police witness, who had not heard this piece of evidence, was also being probed by counsel in trying to build up the picture of the great heat generated. Counsel commented that the heat was so fierce that the dog had to leave in a hurry.

'Yes, that is correct, My Lord. In fact, the dog didn't want to enter and the handler threw him in, but he didn't stay, however, and did a backward somersault straight out again,' was the helpful and truthful reply.

'Quite understandable under the circumstances,' commented the judge with a kindly smile which was reciprocated by both counsel.

The verdict was obviously correct in law, but was disappointing to those who were there that day and did not have the benefit of hindsight, as did the lawyers and various experts who were present in court. Chief Superintendent Swain summed it up to me the next day when he remarked, 'At least, Doc, we didn't have to buy any wreaths,' a sentiment with which we all concurred.

5

NERO:
POLICE DOG SUPERSTAR

Soon after moving into the countryside, we decided that the new house needed a new dog. We already had Jingles, a border collie (and failed sheepdog) given to me by a local farmer, who was a perfect family pet but getting on a bit and suffering from cataracts. My accountant had advised me that if I had a guard dog I could put it down as a tax deductible expense, and Nero came into our lives.

Nero was a champion police dog of the North-amptonshire Police who was in my opinion (and that of his handler Brian Stockwin) retired prematurely from the force when he was still in his prime. Unfortunately, he found difficulty in jumping from any height over three feet and after a hard working day, especially where a lot of jumping or running over uneven ground was involved, he developed a limp. He was diagnosed as suffering from hip dysplasia, a common fault in German shepherd dogs, and at the age of five he was put out to retirement after very distinguished service.

Nobody knew his breeding as he had been found abandoned as a stray in Newcastle. He was taken into care by an animal rescue organisation which in turn gave him to the police training school at Stafford. Brian was sent to train alongside the dog, which returned with his new handler to Northampton. When he retired he had

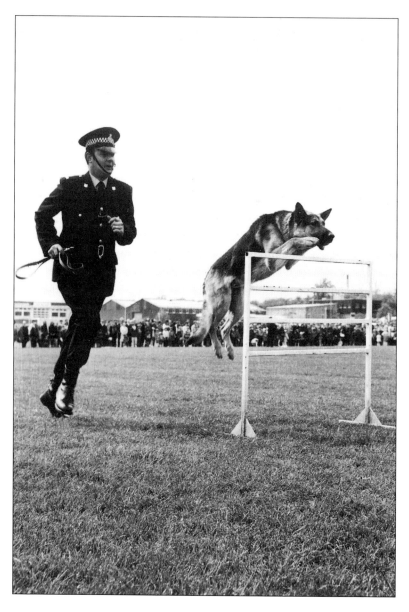

Nero in action with his handler Brian Stockwin.

some 96 arrests to his credit and had found several missing children. During times of what might be called 'civil unrest', for example when the local football team lost at home or the town centre pubs emptied on a Saturday night, the riot van waiting on the market square would not be needed if Nero got there first. Nothing could clear Bridge Street of a crowd quicker than the sight of Nero straining at the leash as Brian fought to keep him at barking distance from the mob.

If you are ever caught by a police dog then stand perfectly still and don't ever try to struggle. The dogs are trained just to hold their jaws in a fixed position and only close them if they feel movement. The old regular villains knew this well but some of the younger ones after a sniff of the barmaid's apron had to find it out by hard experience. I knew from looking at some of Nero's arrests full details of his forensic dentistry long before he came to us.

Nero was a dog with a mind of his own who was always thinking six steps ahead. One of the crowd favourites at police dog displays is when the dog is sent by his handler to retrieve a fresh egg which the handler then breaks into a saucer and gives to the dog as a reward. Nero's version gained him an extra egg. He would retrieve the egg but on the way back would 'accidentally' break it. The crowd would invariably utter a loud gasp of sympathy and genuine disappointment. This would force Brian to put down another egg for retrieval which, with his bushy tail wagging and to roars of approval and cheers from the crowd, Nero would deliver intact.

Although he had very strong jaws, as several local villains could testify, he had a very soft mouth. Like all police dogs when not on duty he lived as a family pet with his handler's family. Brian tells how on one occasion his three year old daughter wandered from home and

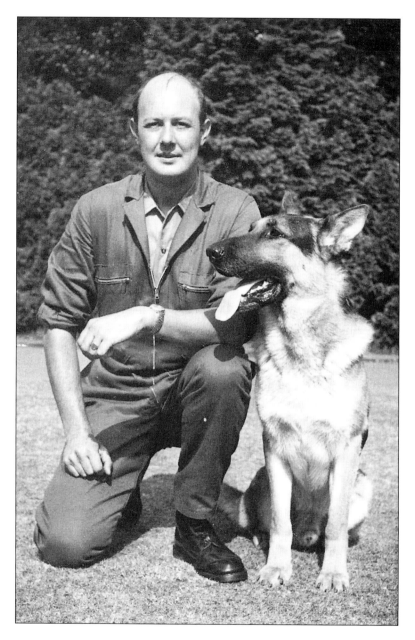

Nero found her in a cornfield, hidden from sight by the tall ripening corn. He gently took her by the arm and led her back to the search party without leaving the slightest bruise or scratch where his teeth had been.

On another occasion they were searching for a shotgun, which Nero was very good at. It is said that a dog's acute sense of smell can detect the scent of the oil in the gun's working parts. Nero frightened Brian by suddenly appearing with the double barrelled gun in his mouth. The normal drill is for the dog to stand and bark, but Nero always had to go one step further.

His independence was also shown when, searching Kettering cemetery for a fugitive, he went into the surrounding hedge and came out with a watering can in his mouth which he laid at Brian's feet, barking excitedly. Brian reasoned that the dog had picked up human scent where someone had recently either kicked or handled the can. As a result a new trail was found and another arrest was added to Nero's tally.

In another incident, four villains were in hiding behind a hedge near Wellingborough and thought they had got away as the searchers passed them by and crossed over to search the other side of the road. However, Nero for no apparent reason suddenly jerked on his lead and pulled Brian in a complete U-turn, returning to the side of the road where they had been a few minutes earlier. Four very surprised and well concealed villains soon felt the steel handcuffs on their wrists, giving themselves up quickly before they also felt Nero's teeth.

He was very protective towards his handler and one Christmas Eve they were patrolling around All Saints church so that the worshippers could attend to their devotions without being disturbed by the drunken revellers coming out of the Bridge Street pubs. After the service a member of the clergy, still dressed in his cassock and surplice, came out to say thank you and, raising his arm, wished Brian a happy Christmas. Only Brian's quick thinking and equally quick reactions saved the clerical arm from being yet another of Nero's trophies.

Nero's arrival at our house after his retirement was like a military operation. The van pulled up in the drive and Nero was taken into the paddock where my son James, who was still at the local village school, was introduced. Sergeant Ramsey supervised as first Brian and then James put the dog through the normal sequence of commands. We were warned that the word we must never use in the hearing of the dog was 'get'.

After an hour or so when we were all at ease with our new pet and guard dog, Brian and the Sergeant took the van down to the bottom of the village where they waited on the radio in case I called for help. None was needed, and putting Nero in the back of the Land Rover we went off to the local pub, where he was left in the vehicle for the local populace to inspect while we enjoyed a drink. One or two commented that the Land Rover was in perfectly good hands, as the dog would not let them get anywhere near it. Then came our first test. When we went to get in, we weren't allowed near it either.

I had a brainwave. We would open the door and let the dog out. James could then walk him home using the drill he had learned from Brian. The exit as per the dog training manual was perfect and with the dog walking to heel in regulation style, James set off home.

Then I suddenly remembered that someone had told me that the dogs were trained so that when they were left in charge of a vehicle they would let no one enter until they were first let out. Their handler opened the driver's door, any passengers were put in and then the dog got back in. Finally, the driver was allowed in and could drive off. As we passed them at the bottom of the village green I stopped, told James to put the dog in the back, then jump in himself. We proceeded without further incident.

On arrival at home there was a perfect dismount by all parties and the dog went ahead of us into the back kitchen. Brian had said this was a good habit, especially if we were coming back to an empty house when there might be burglars inside. Well, as it happened we had had an intruder. The local butcher had been and left the Sunday joint on the kitchen table. Nero was in like a shot and before we realised it the meat was on the floor and the flesh rapidly stripped off the bone. Nobody could or would interfere, and it was obvious that this Sunday's lunch would be at the pub.

As a guard dog Nero was worth his weight in gold and well deserving of his Inland Revenue status as a tax deductible expense. At that time chemists' shops were being burgled all over town by young people involved in the up and coming drugs scene, which although a feature of the larger towns and cities had until then not really been felt in the provincial towns. As we all know, this was to change quickly and today there is no part of the country which is not affected. It has been estimated that between 80 to 90 per cent of the country's crime is drug related.

In rural areas doctors have a dispensary on the premises and carry quite a stock of drugs, so it was not surprising that all the neighbouring surgeries had also been broken into. Mine never was and on seeing a young drug addict in the cells who was quite well known to both me and the police (being such a regular customer that he earned me as much as some of my better off private patients), I asked him why my house had been spared a visit.

65

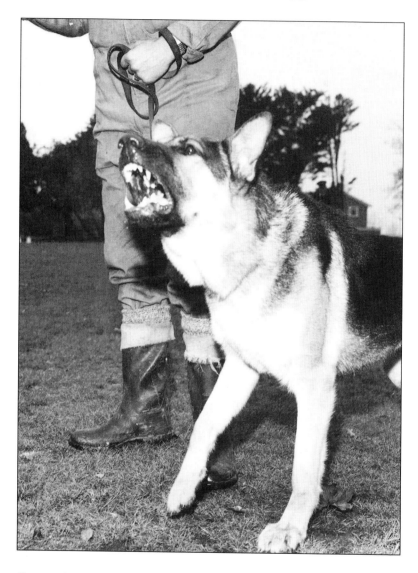

One word we were warned never to use in Nero's hearing was 'Get' – many a villain had found out the hard way to stand perfectly still when caught by Nero.

'Well, Doc,' he replied, 'you've always been good to us and we just wouldn't think about it.'

Then after a pause, when he saw the cynical look in my eyes, 'Also that dog of yours. We remember Nero when that Stockwin had him. He told us that if he bites he never lets go until his teeth meet in the middle. The worst thing is that where the other dogs go for your arm, Nero goes for your ——!'

Needless to say, I encouraged this dog section mythology, which did in fact have some basis in truth. Time and repeated telling of the tale in police canteens over the county had merely introduced some slight exaggeration over the years.

It was at a public relations display when all that was best in the Northamptonshire Police was on view to the local populace. This included Nero and friends. It was a hot day and both dogs and handlers went for fluid replacement in the refreshment tent. When their display started they could not find the runner (the man the dogs chase and grab by his well padded arm) so a fit young cadet was volunteered by his colleagues. He was very realistic in playing the part, for the dog, mistaking the reluctant 'villain' for the real thing, acted accordingly. After the command 'Get' the dog caught up with him and in just a few seconds his teeth had sunk into the seat of the runner's jeans, before Brian could shout the relevant command to disengage.

Nero had completely ignored the padded arm he was meant to seize and had gone for the nearest presenting part of the 'villain's' anatomy. As the news spread to the local criminals, this story became slightly altered. I think the wish was father to the thought as the cadet later became a very active detective officer and a scourge to participants in the Northampton drugs scene.

Nero was quite a character. My daughter had a pet

rabbit named Peter. As a countryman I am well aware that 'Nature is red in tooth and claw', but it did require some tact and a few little white lies to convince my three year old daughter that Peter had run off to see his friends in the next field. A ruse that was nearly ruined when the wretched dog dug up the hastily buried remains, which were then interred deeply in the manure heap. My conscience did prick when for quite some time afterwards she would go into the back field and report sightings.

After the rabbit, the chickens were the target and at first I blamed one of the local foxes. I could find no forensic evidence of the crime, which is unusual for once foxes gain entry to a chicken run they will normally slaughter all the birds and leave them scattered at the scene. Then one afternoon I spotted Nero slinking away from the chicken run with a hen in his mouth.

I decided the way to cure him, which had been related to me by a Cumbrian hill farmer and guaranteed to work, was to tie the corpse to the back of Nero's neck with a piece of strong binder twine. The dog was then to be shut in a stable and left for a week with just a bucket of water. The stench of the decomposing body would act as aversion therapy (as the psychiatrists would call it) and the dog would never look at another chicken.

This was the theory and I followed the instructions as described. After three hours I decided just to check all was well and opened the top half of the stable door to take a little peep. There was Nero sitting up wagging his bushy tail on the stable floor with what can only be described as a smile on his canine face. The only trace of the chicken was a leg with claw attached on a piece of binder twine hanging round his neck like a crucifix. After that we agreed he could have the occasional chicken, just now and again, but his supplies soon ran out after one of the Pytchley foxes took the lot.

That was the only time Nero's vigilance was found wanting and I consoled myself with the fact that the following season we had several good runs on foxes from Creaton Cover, to whom no doubt I had been the munificent benefactor.

Nero's hip dysplasia unfortunately progressed to the stage where he could hardly walk. He used to spend more and more time in the stable, on a comfortable bed of straw alongside Ebony at night, and in the day if the weather was kind enough would crawl up to the paddock gate. Here he would lie in the sun, giving tongue every now and again with a gentle bark or two to let us know that in the paddock 'all was well'. If there were intruders, animal or human, the old bark would soon change. Although he could hardly move, tinkers and itinerant traders were not to know this and rapidly passed us by.

In his heyday he started the day by chasing the horse around the paddock until the horse's hoof made it plain that the game had gone on long enough. The horse was luckily not one which kicked hard and hoof-to-eye coordination was rather slow, so rarely were the kicks more than glancing blows. However, one morning I heard the bark suddenly change into a loud yelp and saw Nero doing a backward somersault over the water trough. He was none the worse for his experience and continued to perform every morning until his legs gave up. Even then, as Ebony passed him by the paddock gate, he would give a little bark and she would gently touch him with her hoof as if to say, 'We're all getting older but there's life in the old dog yet.'

I decided eventually that the kindest thing was to put him to sleep in the stable. After taking advice, I gave Nero his evening meal, a tin of dog food as usual, but into it I packed 20 capsules of sodium amytal. In humans the fatal dose in some cases is as low as five capsules, but when I looked in the next morning Nero was sitting up wagging his tail, obviously not in any pain and feeling the benefit of a good night's sleep. I rang the vet and he told me to repeat the exercise, then when the dog was asleep he would come and give an injection. This was done the next day, the blow being softened a little when John took the opportunity to examine the mare and confirm she was in foal.

Sixteen years have passed since Nero's demise, aged nine, but he is still talked about at police reunions and other gatherings where former police colleagues reminisce.

6

IN
THE WITNESS BOX

In general doctors are listened to and the public, especially their patients, accepts their opinions without question. How different when they go to court, expecting to tell the truth, the whole truth and nothing but the truth. They do not realise that lawyers are not interested in the truth but only in Justice. To put it another way, the lawyer is only interested in winning the case for their client.

In criminal cases, with which I was mostly involved, it is the duty of the prosecution to prove the guilt of the accused beyond reasonable doubt. It is not up to the accused to prove his or her innocence. Any doubts that can be fed to the good citizens of the county, or the twelve of them required to sit in judgement, are therefore fair game and medical evidence provides plenty of scope for confusing the jury.

Defence counsel, it is said, work on the principle:

When the law is against you, use the facts,
When the facts are against you, use the law,
When both the facts and the law are against you,
Then attack the expert!

Understandably many doctors do not like going to court and in my practice my partners were more than

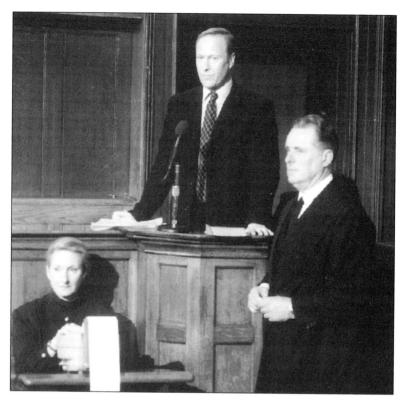

Cross examination is formidable even to the best prepared. Nigel Le Vaillant as Dr Dangerfield stands in what has been described as 'the loneliest place on earth'. A barrister colleague who looked at this photograph and actually saw the relevant episode describes Dangerfield as the perfect medical witness. He is dressed appropriate to the occasion and out of respect to the Court. His body language shows him to be at ease but not 'easy'. He has good eye contact. He thinks and pauses when answering questions, he replies honestly and if he doesn't know, he says so. This is most disarming to a barrister who is trying to draw a doctor outside his field of competence.

Finally he addresses his replies to the jury who come to regard him as a kind and considerate doctor whom they would dearly love to see at the foot of their bed if they are ever taken ill! (*BBC Picture Publicity*) happy for me to take on any case where a court appearance might be a possible outcome, willingly taking on my surgeries and home visits if it meant they would be spared a day in court. It was an arrangement I was quite content with and in return I paid my medico-legal fees into the practice. I enjoyed going to court to escape the trivia of general practice and to relish intellectual debate with the lawyers, some of whom are now among my best friends. I admire the way they are able to read through and assimilate vast bundles of documents and ask the most probing questions, then discard it all and learn a completely different set of facts for the next trial.

Cross-examination is always formidable even to the best prepared and most experienced witness. I still enter the witness box with a little anxiety and concern, rather like an actor going on stage. You are on your own. The witness box can be a very lonely place, but there is great satisfaction to be had if you have given a good performance! The main thing to remember is that the questions are not asked on a personal basis and at the end of the day, lawyers are only doing their best for their client, as is their duty. One's reputation as an expert witness is gained and maintained if you are seen to be strictly non-partisan, acting as a witness for the court rather than the side that called you.

In one case a deputy police surgeon had examined a prisoner after a vigorous arrest following his violent reaction to being invited to assist the 'Old Bill' with their enquiries. The prisoner was a well known villain with several convictions involving drugs and violence, who was also employed as a part-time bouncer at a night club.

It is very tempting as a doctor to believe all that the patient tells you. This is all very well in general practice, but as a police surgeon you must believe nobody (including the police) until after you have looked at the injuries and marks of violence, if any. Then the examiner asks himself if his findings are consistent with the facts he has been told. Do they corroborate any allegations that have been made?

In this case, the prisoner – a six foot three, 17 stone, heavyweight champion type – had a few minor grazes on his body and some linear marks on his back and his right forehead, which he claimed were due to the use of unreasonable force during his arrest (when he offered considerable resistance). My deputy had declared in the written police statement that the injuries were consistent with being beaten by a truncheon, and eventually the case came to a civil action in which the Chief Constable was sued for damages. As the senior police surgeon I had the unenviable task of appearing in court against my colleague and rebutting the evidence to be given on behalf of the plaintiff.

There was no doubt that the good doctor had leaned over backwards to be fair to the then prisoner but had been completely 'conned' in attributing his very minor injuries to a police beating up. There were no proper measurements and certain phrases in the statement showed definite bias on the part of the doctor, which unfortunately came out in court.

The salient points of the doctor's evidence, emphasised by the plaintiff's counsel, were that the marks on the prisoner's head were almost certainly due to a cylindrical object such as a truncheon, and that it was possible to have truncheon marks on the scalp without *any* skin splitting. This is something I have never seen, as on the scalp the skin is stretched directly over the cranium with no underlying connective tissue. The result is that blows that in other regions would produce only bruises, where there is sufficient subdermal tissue to absorb the shock, invariably produce splitting of the skin on the scalp.

Cross-examination by the defence was designed to demonstrate the doctor's inexperience and bias in favour of the plaintiff: 'You are only a deputy police surgeon, and I presume you do not have the experience of your principal?'

'Obviously,' was the only possible reply.

This is the usual belittling approach, used particularly on young doctors at the start of their career. It happens, however, at the other end of the scale too. Mr W. Clegg QC was once very quick to remind me in the most admiring tones that I was on the verge of retirement. I am sure he meant it in a complimentary sense, as we had worked together in the past, but it was also a gentle way of telling the jury that I might be a little past it. Witnesses should not take such remarks to heart as they are not meant to be personal but are designed to unsettle them or at best, from the lawyer's point of view, to get them to lose their temper.

'Did you measure the distance between the parallel red marks on the scalp which you refer to as "tramlines" in your statement?' the cross-examination went on.

'No, I did not.'

'Would you call that a comprehensive examination for this type of case?'

'Yes.'

'In your original statement you said the parallel lines were consistent with the sole of a boot. Have you thought of any other explanation, Doctor?'

'On further reflection I consider them more likely to be from a cylindrical object like a truncheon.'

Here the barrister was using sarcasm in his cross-examination technique but the doctor maintained his professional dignity in reply, although not very convincingly. The cross-examination proceeded as various alternative and in some cases more credible explanations were offered which of course the doctor had to concede. The original statement had now taken on a completely different meaning and Counsel sat down with a satisfied smile on his face.

It was my turn next on behalf of the defendant, ie the Chief Constable, who although he had never met the plaintiff was as chief officer defending on behalf of his force. I suspected that opposing counsel would make a point to the jury inferring that the title 'police surgeon' meant I was the coppers' doctor and that my evidence would therefore be biased in their favour.

'How long have you been a police surgeon?'

'Thirty four years.' Anticipating the line he was going to follow I continued, 'But I do other medico-legal work as well and have a private practice.'

'But Northamptonshire Police are your main employers?'

'No, sir. They provide less than a third of my total income. As you are aware, I spend a great portion of my professional time advising barristers and solicitors on medical matters.'

That line of questioning quickly ceased as to take it further might produce an unexpected answer and damage his case. This was followed by various probing questions on each individual bruise and graze, suggesting it was possible or even highly probable that they had been made by police batons, knuckles or boots. The routine answers which Counsel expected and got, conceded the possibility but I added, '...although exceedingly unlikely.' At the same time I looked directly at the jury, with a slight lifting of the eyebrow to stress the word 'unlikely'. The appropriate body language at the appropriate time can work wonders with a jury.

The final question was, 'Don't you think, Doctor, with all your years of experience, that in arresting this citizen the police officers went just a little bit over the top?'

My answer: 'No, the injuries are consistent with reasonable force being used against a strong, powerfully built man who we have heard landed on the floor and resisted with vigour, efforts to put him in the van.'

The final outcome was that the plaintiff lost his case for damages on the alleged assault but was awarded minor damages on a technical breach of arresting procedure which was admitted by the defendant.

It is useful to understand the games lawyers play. Remember, no good lawyer ever asks a question to which they do not know the answer and one of the objects of cross-examination is to try to lead the doctor outside his field of competence. So many young police surgeons fall for the pleasant preamble, 'I am only a simple layman, I wonder if you could explain in simple terms that myself and the jury can understand...?' or, 'I know you do not usually work in this field but I wonder if you might help us on this small point...?' Young doctors whose egos are temporarily inflated by this implied respect for their medical knowledge fall easily into the trap of going outside their field of competence, like lambs being led to slaughter.

It is always an education to hear the different meanings that lawyers can put on plain English words. Many times my 'opinion' has been referred to as my 'guess or pure conjecture', my 'belief' became 'your theory, Doctor', and to refer to something as unusual or rare was interpreted as 'perplexing'. To say you were convinced brought the rejoinder that you were prejudiced, and if you conceded that something was remotely possible then you had to agree that, 'It's not inconsistent, is it Doctor?'

The most disarming answer to any barrister is 'I don't know', if you can honestly say so. The old adage, 'Stand up, speak up, and shut up' is very true of court appearances. So is the old army rule, 'Time spent in reconnaissance is never wasted', which I obeyed implicitly.

As Shakespeare pointed out, 'All the world's a stage, and all the men and women merely players...' In court however, I always remembered it was a lawyer's stage and I was only there as a guest artist or as part of the backing group for their act. I would leave the humorous remarks and snide comments to the lawyers, but always smiled indulgently, they of course not realising that I had heard it all before. Judicial quips were in a different category and invariably worthy of true recognition, but above all they were never to be upstaged, no matter how tempting.

One young barrister with a Persil-white wig was prolonging his cross-examination of me and prefixing all his questions with, 'Are you not surprised, Doctor?' His Lordship, who I knew was expected at Towcester Races for lunch, eventually spoke from the bench. 'Mr So and So, I have had many long and happy years at the Bar but I have never met a police surgeon who is surprised at anything!'

My cross-examination soon finished and the Judge's horse came in first, I was delighted to hear.

Pathologists, like doctors, sometimes stray outside their field of competence. Our local Home Office pathologist, Dr Peter Andrews from Kettering with whom I had an excellent working relationship for over 20 years, was one day persuaded to advise a local solicitor in the defence of a businessman who was accused of driving while under the influence of alcohol. This was pre-breathalyser, and also in the days of the 'ambush defence' when the defence did not have to disclose expert evidence to the prosecution as they are now obliged to do. Excellent pathologist that Peter was, I knew he had never examined a drunk in charge.

I was not at first involved but on the first day of the trial I received a panic phone call at lunchtime when the prosecution heard that Peter was coming to court in the afternoon. It was apparent that the accused, who operated a dry cleaning shop, was going to claim that the symptoms which had suggested he was drunk were in fact caused by exposure to Trilene fumes at his work. I was asked to come and listen to the evidence and if possible be prepared to go into the witness box to rebut it.

On my way to court I went into the medical room of the Avon Cosmetics factory where I was a part-time medical adviser, and took a very large book off the shelf. It was the size of an old-fashioned family bible but when carried with some difficulty under my arm, the title in gold lettering could be clearly read: *Toxicity of Industrial Solvents*. I had never had the time or need to open it before and to be truthful have never opened it since, but it served me well that afternoon.

As I walked into the foyer of the court I saw Peter standing with the defence counsel and with a smile tapped the book, holding it so he could easily read the title. 'It's all in here, Peter,' I said, then moved off quickly before he could ask to look at it.

Trilene was in fact often used as an anaesthetic, but it had to be administered with great caution as the safety margin between a deep sleep and death was a very thin line. As I think Peter strongly suspected, the amount of Trilene needed to produce the same effects as observed by the police surgeon would have meant the client, if not dead, would hardly have been able to climb into his car, let alone drive it in the manner he was when arrested.

There was a conference between the client, the barrister and Peter. The barrister then walked over to his learned friend for the prosecution and announced that

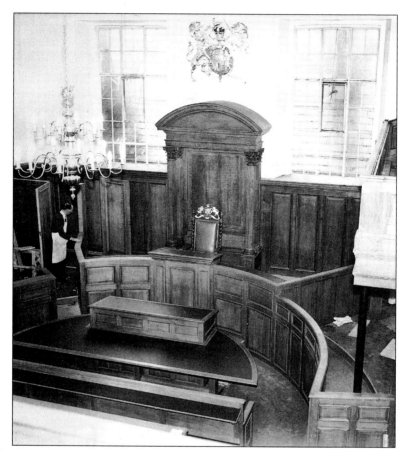

Inside Northampton's historic Crown Court.

the doctors would not be needed as his client was pleading guilty.

Neither of us having anything else to do for the afternoon, Peter and I walked across the road to discuss diverse medico-legal matters in the Barrel Bar just opposite the old Crown Court, in George Row. This magnificent old court building had the Judge's lodgings on one side, a Union Jack flying from the flagpole when a High Court Judge was in residence, and the County Council chamber on the other side.

One feature of Court Number One is that the public gallery is in the balcony, an architectural tradition that is not followed in modern courts. One of the most amusing days I spent in that court was when one of our local young hooligans was accused of causing grievous bodily harm to a police officer – an offence, by the way, which carries a maximum sentence of life imprisonment.

'Big Martin', as he was known, was the police gaoler at Campbell Square. An ex-military policeman standing six foot three inches in his stockinged feet, he was in fact a gentle giant. He did, however, expect respect and good order from the prisoners and discipline was always maintained when he was in charge.

Persistent troublemakers would, as fate and the magistrates decreed, invariably find themselves on their way to the young offenders prison at Glen Parva in the cell van with Martin driving. Rumour had it he had learned to drive in a tank and this was reflected in his gear changing and braking techniques, which tended to hurl the unfortunate prisoners against the sides of the very narrow cubicles in the cell van. One day there was a riot in the cell block which Martin managed to quell almost single-handed, but during the proceedings he received a kick in the testicles from one of the young prisoners, who perhaps could not face another trip to Glen Parva with Martin driving.

The youth was charged and Dr Checka Rao, who had just started as a deputy police surgeon, examined both the prisoner and Martin. He eventually presented the evidence which included a description of the very minor injury to Martin's nether regions. At the time the court rose for lunch, Dr Rao had given his evidence but the

Judge asked if he would make himself available to come back in the afternoon when Martin himself would be in the witness box.

There were only one or two of the local villains sitting in the gallery, but they got the impression that Dr Rao was going to be asked to carry out another intimate examination that afternoon. When the court reconvened after lunch, all the local villains had left the steps of All Saints where they normally bought and sold their drugs, and had crowded into the public gallery. They were most disappointed when the Judge, having ascertained from Martin that he was fully recovered, immediately released Dr Rao from the court. The public gallery soon emptied to the smiles of judge, jury and counsel – with a bemused Martin standing in the box wondering why he was losing his fan club in one mass exodus.

The carved woodwork in the two old courtrooms, especially in Court Number One, is well worth seeing, a credit to Northampton craftsmen of the 19th century and perhaps the century before. Above the witness box in Court Number One is a carved face of the devil. It is said that when a witness told a damnable lie, the devil put out his tongue. Legend has it that this has been seen on several occasions, though I can vouch that it never happened when I was giving evidence. However, one day in the late morning I was sitting in the seats normally reserved for the probation officers. The sun coming through the skylight was shining on the devil's face in such a way that it cast a shadow which made it look as if the tongue was protruding. Have I at long last solved a psychic phenomenon?

7

A CASE OF CHILD POISONING

The syndrome of Munchausen by Proxy is now well documented and a recognised element in the study of child abuse. Munchausen Syndrome is named after the German Baron Munchausen who was a notorious raconteur and famous for telling tall stories. In medical parlance it refers to those patients who travel from doctor to doctor, or from hospital to hospital inventing false illnesses and suffering all sorts of investigations, even unnecessary operations, in order to get attention. It is deemed to be 'by Proxy' when a parent or other responsible adult uses the illness of a child to gain approval or attention, themselves creating the illness they seem so anxious to alleviate.

It was not generally thought possible in the 1970s, when non-accidental injury to children was beginning to be professionally recognised, that a mother or other caring adult would inflict injury, sometimes life-threatening, on a child in their care in order to gain attention. If it did happen, then it was only because they were clinically insane and could be seen to be so. Events of recent years, however, have shown it can and does occur in persons who suffer a personality disorder – or in old fashioned terms are clever, devious and dangerous psychopaths – as was illustrated in the case of the children's nurse, Beverley Allitt.

A case in 1976 which was eventually heard at North-ampton Crown Court illustrated the effectiveness of the liaison scheme established at Northampton General Hospital as a result of the increased awareness of child abuse following the notorious case of Maria Colwell in 1967. As police surgeon, I acted as liaison officer between the medical personnel involved and the police in the detection of a case of child abuse which would probably otherwise have had fatal consequences.

Jeremy (not his real name) was admitted at the age of 15 months having taken four Paramol tablets allegedly left in the house by his maternal grandmother. On admission to Northampton General Hospital he was sleepy but otherwise well. Blood analysis showed a raised para-cetamol level. This was retested the following morning, when it had fallen to an acceptable level as expected. The next day the blood level had fallen almost to zero and it was considered safe to discharge the child home the following day.

The mother, Mrs E, was in fact qualified as a State Registered Nurse and also as a Registered Mental Nurse, but this was not known until the child's second admission, when she told one of the nursing staff. What she did not declare was that she had been removed from the register by the General Nursing Council for larceny of drugs. She had also been put on probation with a condition that she be assessed and receive psychiatric treatment.

Mrs E visited Jeremy, who was perfectly well clinically and was really only being detained in hospital a further day to await the results of liver function tests, which had been carried out as paracetamol is a liver poison. That afternoon however, the child was noticed to be sleepy and 'floppy' after she had gone home.

The next day with the test results reported normal, she

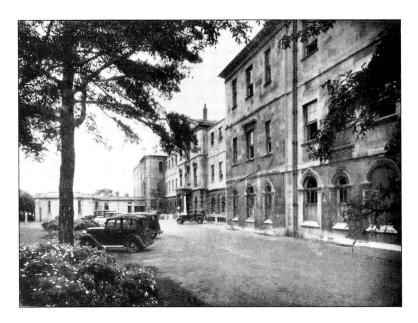

Northampton General Hospital – much as it looked in 1957 when the author arrived for the very first time!

arrived to reluctantly take Jeremy home. She was also coping at home with a six week old baby, but another reason for her reluctance was explained to the ward sister. There had been an older child of Mrs E's first marriage. This child had died at the age of 18 months after a whooping cough injection, when the family were on holiday in a caravan in Cornwall. The child had become fractious, was given paracetamol and 'just faded away' a few hours later following admission to hospital as a suspected case of encephalitis.

The Northampton staff did not know at the time that there had been no post mortem examination and with sympathy accepted the mother's diagnosis, while strongly reassuring her that Jeremy was fit for her to take home. Because of her anxiety they offered to keep him until the next morning. When Mrs E had gone, once more the child was observed to be sleepy with poor muscular tone. Next morning he had fully recovered and was duly collected by his mother.

That evening the GP had a telephone call from Mrs E to say that Jeremy was sleepy, but she had been told to expect this as the child had had a lumbar puncture to exclude any disease of the central nervous system such as encephalitis. She was reassured but told to ring back in a couple of hours if she was still worried. She rang back at 8 pm to say Jeremy had vomited twice and was now so sleepy she could not rouse him. After a home visit, and with nothing on physical examination to explain the child's comatose state, Jeremy was readmitted to hospital. Both parents seemed extremely distressed and concerned for the welfare of the child.

On admission Jeremy was in a very comatosed state with poor respiration. He was put on the cardiac monitor and an intravenous transfusion set up. Blood was taken for drug testing, but though negative for alcohol and barbiturates the blood was not tested for paracetamol at this time. (A sample was held back for further testing if necessary and a few days later when the police had become involved, tests by the Home Office Forensic Science Laboratory showed a very high level of this substance.)

Jeremy recovered quickly that night and the next morning when examined in the presence of his mother was in all respects normal. He objected vigorously and loudly when taken away from her to be examined on the bed. His muscle tone and power were normal and no abnormality was demonstrated in any system. His mother had stayed overnight in the special suite reserved for parents in such circumstances and had generally helped with looking after the child.

She did, however, ask for Epanutin, phenobarbitone and Valium for herself, saying that her doctor prescribed these for epilepsy and she had left her pills at home. The staff were unable to provide Valium and a staff nurse was dispatched to another ward to get some. The nurse was told to make sure that Mrs E took them herself. She didn't, in fact, so a relay of nurses kept her under observation while attending to their other duties. They had already decided amongst themselves that there was 'something odd' going on.

Their vigil was rewarded when Jeremy was seen while being nursed on his mother's lap to be making mouthing movements and grimacing. Sister was told and after consultation with the medical staff the child was taken from his mother and into the treatment room. Here a stomach wash-out was carried out and on analysis this demonstrated the presence of Valium. A blood sample taken at the same time also confirmed the presence of Valium and paracetamol.

After lunch Jeremy walked round the ward with a nurse and Mrs E left the hospital to do some shopping. At this point the story is best unfolded by quoting parts of the statement given to the police by Nurse S, who had spent a considerable time with the mother and child.

'I checked the room and removed anything that baby was using. I removed a feeding bottle with milk in and an empty beaker but left some dirty plates and a beaker on a chair. Mrs E was not on the ward at this time. I then left Baby E with Nurse B and told him to take half-hourly pulses and give drinks which were in the refrigerator.

'About an hour later I was told that the baby had been vomiting. I changed the baby and the bed and noticed the vomit was powdery. I did not suspect anything was wrong so I washed the baby's face and put the clothing out for washing. I noticed that Nurse B had taken the beaker from the room and the contents appeared to be milk that had curdled. He said that Mrs E had returned from the shops and had been holding the baby while he vomited, making the remark, "He always vomits on me."

'I then noticed that there were two brown bags and a paper bag with "Boots" on it in the room. She said she had been out to buy cakes for her husband. The bag marked Boots was inside one of the cake bags which made me suspicious as one does not normally put anything else in the same bag as cakes.'

The statement then went on to say that the nurse talked with Mrs E about her family and the child who had died, eliciting a remark from Mrs E: 'This is just how the other one went.' Nurse S then described how she was nursing Jeremy and remarked to a passing doctor that the baby was 'all floppy' again and unable to sit unaided.

She continued: 'I went for my tea break and cleared out the room leaving only a disposable nappy, hairbrush and his identity band in the room. I left Mrs E and told her to ask a nurse for a drink if she felt Jeremy wanted one. While I was later giving the rest of the children their teas I noticed Mrs E giving Jeremy a drink. I said to someone passing, "Who the hell gave her that drink?" and nobody seemed to know. We discussed it and later when Mrs E left the room I searched and found the beaker on a ledge behind the screen. Mrs E would have had to make a special effort to put the cup where I found it. I took the lid off and saw it contained a clear liquid but I saw some white powdery substance down one side of it. I realised it was not vomit or milk and I tasted it. It was very bitter and salty.

'I found Nurse Y and asked her to look at the beaker and what she thought should be done. Nurse Y tasted it and immediately said, "My God, it's caked with something like phenobarbitone or something. What's she trying to do to that child?" Staff Nurse M then called the doctor. I went back to the cubicle where the baby was and looked in the two cake bags. I found the cakes but not the Boots bag. I then remembered Mrs E used the mother and baby room so I checked in there and found in one of the disposal bins a screwed up Boots bag. I opened the bag and removed an empty bottle which had according to the label contained twelve paracetamol tablets.'

Police enquiries subsequently confirmed that Mrs E had that afternoon bought twelve soluble paracetamol tablets at Boots. The shop assistant clearly remembered her as no other similar tablets had been asked for that day.

Back at the hospital the doctors gently expressed their concern to his parents about Jeremy and also the six week old baby at home. The husband at first was very hostile and would not believe that his wife could do anything like what was being alleged.

I was contacted while this was going on and warned the appropriate police officer. A three-sided telephone conversation took place between the consultant, myself and the Detective Chief Inspector, when it was decided that immediate action was necessary. Fortunately, of the various samples that had been taken for analysis during both the first and second admissions sufficient residues remained for me to collect and send to the Home Office Forensic Science Laboratory at Huntingdon. The results of the hospital were all confirmed.

Mrs E threatened suicide so she was taken into custody, mainly for her own safety, and I arranged a consultation with a consultant psychiatrist as an emergency. I knew he had considerable experience in forensic psychiatry. He reported: 'My feeling is that she is a highly immature and devious personality. This concept is a difficult one to argue convincingly as it is based on impression rather than concrete evidence.' However, he went on, further enquiries needed to be made into her actions. 'There will come a time when we shall have to decide whether she looks after her children at all.'

It was a valuable emergency assessment and I duly made further enquiries into her medical history, with her fully informed consent, given on the advice of her solicitor. My relationship with Mrs E while she was in my care for two days was excellent and she was bailed while enquiries continued. Her own GP and the Health Visitor had been made aware of events and the children were being looked after by relatives.

I scrutinised letters from hospitals all over the UK, the main areas of her travels having found her attending hospitals (on her own behalf) in London, Glasgow, Suffolk, Essex and Northamptonshire. The most common diagnosis was hysterical psychopathy, although various other labels were suggested by the woman herself and eagerly adopted by some of the many doctors whose paths she had crossed (e.g. epilepsy, blackouts, encephalitis, migraine, Royal Free disease, and other forms of a condition known as neurasthenia). Barbiturates featured prominently in her therapy. She could certainly be considered an unusual presentation of the Munchausen Syndrome.

It was on the advice of the Director of Public Prosecutions that she was charged with two offences of wilful neglect in administering noxious substances to her son Jeremy, to which she pleaded guilty. The start of the trial was delayed because she became pregnant and was subsequently delivered of another child. All her children were taken into care by the local authority. Mrs E was made the subject of a Hospital Order without limit of time under Section 60 of the Mental Health Act.

The case proved the effectiveness of the inter-agency approach to the investigation of suspected child abuse in Northampton, an initiative that later became adopted nationwide. After the case was concluded, the Judge made some very complimentary remarks about the way it had been handled from the outset by all those involved. He added, 'I think I must also commend the medical staff concerned because they obviously had their wits very much about them as far as the welfare of the child was concerned, coupled with, as far as I can see, commendable tact in dealing with this unfortunate lady.' It also demonstrated the useful role a police surgeon could play as liaison officer between Medicine and Law, especially on a local level where he has a foot in both camps.

8

MURDER:
THE WARDELL CASE

I am often asked, 'What is your most famous murder case?' (The questioner really means 'most infamous case'!) Or, which case do I remember most clearly? The answer is that there is not one particular case that stands out in my mind – all murders are tragic and upsetting. Every case is different, but each one requires the same amount of concentration and forensic expertise.

A good example was the successful prosecution of Gordon Wardell at Oxford Crown Court, for the murder of his wife Carol in September 1994. Mr Justice Cresswell's remarks in sentencing him to life imprisonment were very brief and to the point:

'You are an extremely dangerous, evil and devious man. This murder was an outrage ... Take him down.'

Carol Wardell was manageress of the Nuneaton branch of the Woolwich Building Society. Her body was found in a lay-by near Coventry after, Gordon Wardell claimed, she and her husband were attacked at home on Sunday, 11th September 1994.

Wardell described to the police how a gang of three men with clown mask disguises broke into their bungalow. They punched him in the stomach (one punch, he told the police) and then put a pad soaked in some volatile anaesthetic such as chloroform over his face,

92

which made him unconscious. He claimed to remember nothing more until next morning when he heard the milkman and awoke to find himself tightly bound in a steel box-like frame used to put rubbish sacks in. He had struggled to escape but was unable to do so as his hands and feet were tightly bound with thick plastic industrial ties. He was eventually found by police who came to the bungalow after discovering Carol's body in the lay-by.

The building society branch had been entered and £14,000 taken from the safe, opened with Carol's key. On the floor was one of Carol's slippers.

Wardell was rushed to hospital in the care of two CID officers, who remained with him during and after examination, where nothing of significance was found. His reaction on being informed of the death of his wife was described as 'odd' – he just asked whether she had been sexually assaulted.

Gordon Wardell's behaviour that day and the day following showed an exaggeration of his alleged shock and pain. This was seen nationally when he made a television appearance in a wheelchair, which he insisted he needed despite reassurance by the medical staff and to the surprise of the two police officers who had been sitting with him. He made a tearful request for anyone with information to contact the police. Audience reaction generally (and not only from sceptical policemen) was that he was performing an act worthy of an Equity card.

Detective Superintendent Tony Bayliss had a fine team of CID officers around him for this case, backed up by a well trained HOLMES team. The latter is now a feature of all murder enquiries and was set up after the Yorkshire Ripper enquiry. The letters stand for Home Office Local Major Enquiry Service and every force throughout the UK has trained a number of officers and civilians to undertake this role.

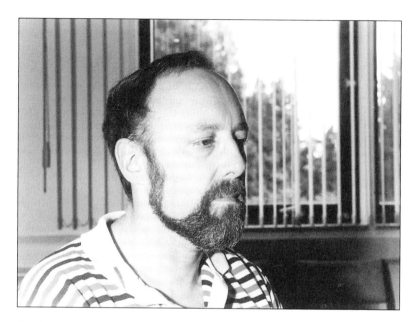

Gordon Wardell

Dr Paul Miller, the local police surgeon, had done the initial examination of Wardell. His painstaking recording of the injuries (some of them very minute), together with the initial and subsequent photography, were a great help to me when I was called in as a consultant to advise on the interpretation of the injuries. This was a role I had performed for several forces quite regularly over the years following my appointment in 1970 as a part-time Honorary Clinical Assistant to the Department of Forensic Medicine at the London Hospital Medical College.

When Detective Superintendent Tony Bayliss met me in the Incident Room at Nuneaton, he had already received some useful information. The prostitutes of Coventry apparently knew Wardell well, as over the years he had used their services often. This information could not be given to the jury at the subsequent trial as in the event of a successful prosecution it might have been held by the Court of Appeal to be prejudicial. However, it was of great investigative value, as were many other titbits of information phoned in after Wardell's television appearance.

Tony gave me a very good briefing, including the report of the pathologist that Carol had died from asphyxia due to strangulation. The information on Wardell was followed by a grim but smiling reminder: 'We don't believe he is telling the truth.'

He said no more, as it would have been most unprofessional to do so. Any forensic doctor must approach a case with an open mind. There is an old forensic aphorism that: 'Things are not always what they first seem.' Another stresses the need to keep an open mind: 'The human mind is like a parachute – it works better when it is open.' I made a conscious effort as I realised it was now all down to me. My antennae of suspicion were certainly switched on – like everyone else who watched Wardell's appearance on television, I felt there was something not quite right – but my mind was open.

The story of the anaesthetic certainly didn't ring true. I well remembered from my days as an SHO anaesthetist (incidentally, often using the old 'rag and bottle' technique) how difficult it was to get the patient to sleep and then to keep him asleep. Most surgeons I was detailed to work for made comments to the effect that if the patient could keep awake, I shouldn't have found it too difficult! I therefore felt that it was extremely doubtful that Wardell could have been given an anaesthetic so successfully that it caused his long period of unconsciousness.

I also took with a pinch of salt that one of the gang members had punched him a violent blow in the stomach. On examination later there were merely several bruises across the front of his abdomen typical of 'pinch bruises', often seen in non-accidental injuries to children but in this case almost certainly self-inflicted.

The bruises on his arms (which the day after the incident Paul Miller had thought might be consistent with grasp marks) had by the time I saw them developed properly. They were rectangular and consistent more with contact with a blunt surface such as the edge of furniture than with grasp marks made by an assailant. They too, therefore, could have been self-inflicted.

From enquiries made I was able to build up a picture which, again from an investigative point of view, was quite useful, especially when complemented by the information provided by the prostitutes and the opinion of Paul Britton, a well known forensic psychologist who gave us a very good psychological profile of Wardell. None of this could be used in evidence, but as bits of the investigative jigsaw they contributed to the final picture of the murderer.

In 1970 at Winson Green Prison Wardell had been seen by Dr Robert Bluglass, a forensic psychiatrist of some repute, when serving a sentence following a sexual attack at knifepoint in which the victim was almost killed when he stabbed her twice in the neck. He was a 17 year old schoolboy at the time and had lured the wife of one of his teachers into a wood on the pretext of showing her a rare plant. He was charged with attempted murder but this was reduced to causing grievous bodily harm and he served four years in prison, including Grendon psychiatric prison, but he did not really open up to the staff there so, as events were to show, he did not benefit from his time in that establishment.

Wardell's home background was interesting. He was the only child of a college lecturer and schoolmistress mother. She was said to be very domineering and taught

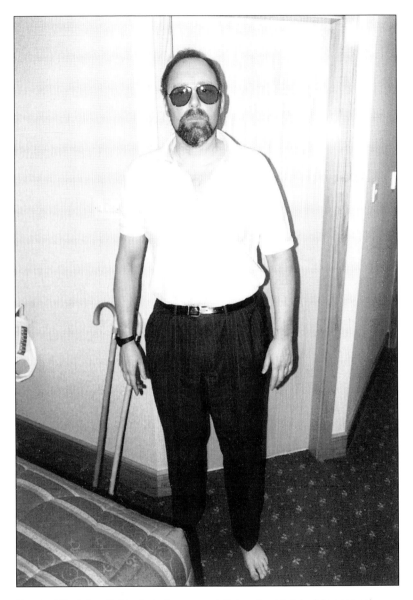

Gordon Wardell, with his dark glasses and sticks after his television appeal.

young Gordon to cook, knit and sew, subjects she taught at her school. She closely controlled his friends and activities as he grew up.

His marriage to Carol appeared to the outside world to be perfectly steady. They regularly enjoyed overseas holidays together and would often be accompanied by Carol's widowed mother. Even after the crime he gave support to his mother-in-law, walking arm in arm with her at the funeral.

After his wife's murder, Wardell stayed with relatives of Carol's at a secret address to escape the Press and it was there that I was taken to examine him a week later. He was fully co-operative but I got the feeling that he was very much on the defensive. He had a limp and sweaty handshake, wore dark glasses in the house and leaned heavily on his walking stick. He moved with what I thought were exaggerated movements to convey the discomfort he was suffering. My 'gut feelings', however, were not evidence that would stand up in court and all this could easily be explained as a post-traumatic stress reaction to the ordeal he had been through and grief at the loss of his wife.

However, there were physical findings originally noted by Dr Miller, painstakingly recorded on the body chart diagrams and photographed daily as they developed. Apart from the abdominal bruising (which was not consistent with having been caused by a single blow from a fist as alleged by Wardell), the arm bruising was patterned and consistent with self infliction. The injuries which carried most weight in my mind were the tiny puncture-type scratches only 2mm long distributed over Wardell's hands and wrists, noted by Dr Miller on his initial examination and still present when I examined Wardell a week later. They were in my opinion caused by Carol's fingernails as she tried to release the pressure when his hands tightened around her neck.

Gordon Wardell was finally charged with the murder of his wife, Carol. At the trial both Dr Miller and I underwent prolonged cross-examination from Mr W. Clegg QC, as did all the other important police witnesses, but at the end of the day the jury returned a guilty verdict.

Wardell still protests his innocence of the crime. An eminent forensic psychologist has expressed the view that he is unlikely to ever admit to his guilt as this appears to have been a typical anger-retaliation murder, often seen in cases where men have been female-dominated, especially in their youth. Such men cannot accept responsibility for their crime or even for the fact they have done wrong.

There is still a mystery to be solved, as the police have never traced the £14,000 stolen from the building society the night Carol Wardell died. Was it hidden away, or used to pay off debts, perhaps blackmail? Or was it given to one of the prostitutes Gordon Wardell associated with? One day, perhaps, we shall learn the whole truth.

9

DANGERFIELD
PEBBLE MILL'S OWN POLICE
SURGEON

During my time as Honorary Secretary to the Association, when I also acted as press secretary, my duties had on several occasions found me attending the news studios at BBC Pebble Mill. Little did I think I would ever end up in the Drama department! Some people spend the whole of their lives trying to get inside the BBC halls of fame (provided they can find a parking place), but I landed there by pure accident.

It was in 1995, when I was still President of the Association of Police Surgeons, that my children informed me a new television series called *Dangerfield* was starting, all about the adventures of a police surgeon, played by Nigel le Vaillant. The central character was a general practitioner in the ancient city of Warwick, who like myself in my earlier days found it hard to balance the demands of police work with his practice, much to the chagrin of his long-suffering partners.

The first few episodes were written by the author Don Shaw and based on the experiences of his friend, Dr Mick Bletcher. Mick had by then retired from his general practice, which had included many years of yeoman service to the Derbyshire Constabulary. He had also been a stalwart member of the Association and like me, many of his friends who were watching those early episodes were delighted to see his name on the credits as medical adviser.

'Mick's new programme', as we called it, soon became a talking point amongst our members. Despite a few technical errors such as the Land Rover changing its wheels during the programme, and a 'corpse' who closed his eyes while being confirmed dead, the technical side of the work of a police surgeon was well portrayed – although dramatic licence necessitated a rather large workload for rural Warwickshire!

One member, however, strongly criticised Dangerfield's wearing apparel, and found him guilty of so many breaches of procedure and ethics that he felt he should register for the National Training Course without delay. I was at the time joint director of this course, which it was intended all new police surgeons should attend on appointment. It was held at the National Training Centre for Scientific Support to Crime Investigation at Harperley Hall, a beautiful country house in the middle of County Durham. It trained not only police surgeons but also fingerprint experts, photographers, and forensic experts from all over the UK. A department of the Durham Constabulary, it issues diplomas from the University of Durham, so there is an academic aura about the place.

Then in one episode Dangerfield went to court dressed in a pair of jeans and a sweatshirt. I had been in close touch with Mick, discussing what had gone out in each episode and keeping him up to date with the latest developments in the service, and Mick told me that he had made it known to the powers-that-be that our hero was improperly dressed for the occasion, but to no avail. With the backing of Mick and several senior members of the Association, I therefore wrote to the producer, congratulating him on the series so far but offering a few

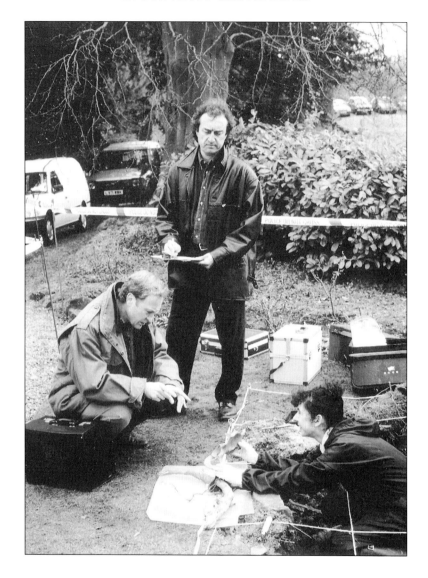

constructive suggestions which I hoped he would find helpful.

As a result, I was asked to help with the production as assistant to Mick. This was an excellent arrangement as Mick went out on location and I would receive copies of the scripts as well, so the two of us could cross-check with each other before giving the green light to the script editor to go ahead. We both felt this was important, not only to check medical accuracy but also to confirm that the content was credible for a professional police surgeon.

Problems with a script would only arise when things were put in by the writers that would not happen in real life. A certain amount of dramatic and artistic licence is necessary, but not too often and not too much or the whole story would lose credibility. Thousands of police officers watch the series, as well as doctors and nurses – and police surgeons! If both Mick and I felt that something needed to be altered, a compromise solution was invariably worked out in the early stages in discussion with the script editor and author. For each episode there was first an initial script on white paper, and revisions to the script followed at intervals on different coloured paper, until we eventually finished up with a pink 'rehearsal script'. Even when it came to filming, the director would make alterations if he was not happy with

Nigel Le Vaillant as Dr Paul Dangerfield 'discovers a body' in the second series. Even small pieces of human remains can give a vast amount of forensic information. This is actually part of a female pelvic girdle from which the victim's age and other information can be obtained. Forensic anthropologists (anatomists) and forensic dentists are increasingly being called upon to help pathologists and the West murder enquiry in Gloucester in 1994 brought their work to the attention of the general public. (*BBC Picture Publicity*)

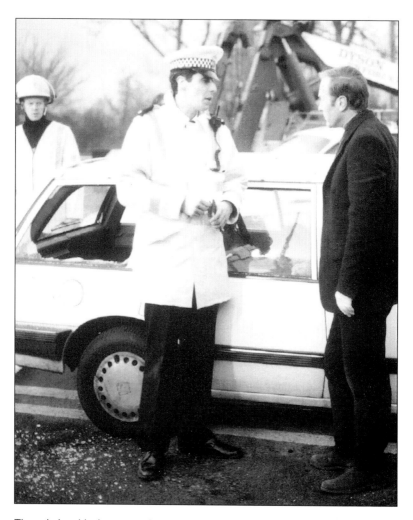

The relationship between the police and the police surgeon is an important element in the series. This scene depicts a fatal road traffic accident – unfortunately a regular occurrence for traffic officers where the attendance of a police surgeon is often required. These are stressful occasions for all involved. Post incident debriefing also includes post traumatic stress counselling. In Northamptonshire the force welfare department often includes the medical officer as part of the team. (*BBC Picture Publicity*)

something, usually deleting rather than adding, as one cannot expect the actors to learn new lines on location. Time and money were also factors, bearing in mind that a day's shooting can cost between £18,000 and £25,000.

Towards the end of the second series Mick wanted to go to Canada to visit his family, and I took over the location work as well. A new producer was appointed for the third series and he asked me to continue. I now had Dr Peter Green to help me. Peter and I were very old friends, having served for many years on various committees together. At one point he had appeared in a BBC2 programme called *40 Minutes*, which spent a night following him around on call in the Brixton area. It was my suggestion he be approached, as the area he works in is probably the busiest in the country, and when he is on call there is very little chance he will crawl into bed until the dawn is breaking.

To a doctor whose professional life has been well planned and organised, with meticulous attention to detail, it is both a culture shock and a fast learning experience to find oneself in the middle of what at first sight appears absolute chaos. Filming is in fact as meticulous in its planning, attention to detail and organisation as any surgical operation. The difference is that the place is teeming with people carrying anything from clipboards and pieces of equipment to mugs of tea – but they all know what they have to do and are always to be found in the right place at the right time when the cameras roll. This is essential if the director sitting in his studio chair, his eyes flitting from the action to the monitor and with the continuity girl at his side taking copious notes and timings, is to get through the day's tasks before they 'wrap up' at the end of a very full day.

For the electricians and scenery shifters, the make-up girls and costume department, the day starts an hour or

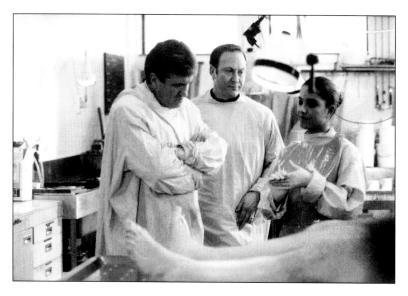

The autopsy – CID coming to terms with the finding. (*BBC Picture Publicity*)

so before shooting and ends an hour or two after it finishes. For these and other support staff a 16 hour day is the norm. For the actors it is also a long day but most of it is spent waiting about to be called on set. The stars have a personal caravan but the back-ups and extras wait in what is euphemistically called the green room. Here many sit and chat, while some bring hobbies such as needlework or painting to while away the time. As all these people require food the mobile caterers provide meals in a converted double decker bus. This becomes a focal point for us all to get together at least three times a day, starting with breakfast at 0700 hours for those on call. Everyone works hard, but there is a marvellous team spirit so the time soon passes.

At the end of shooting a series feelings are mixed. There is satisfaction and pride at a job well done but also sadness at saying goodbye to friends who are going to pastures new. Quite a few are not sure where they are going next but an air of optimism pervades as they know that 'something will turn up'. It is truly amazing that actors and show business folk in general seem to be able to accept as a matter of course that long periods of their working lives will be spent 'resting'. Although any conversation sooner or later turns to their agents and their next jobs it certainly doesn't seem to worry them.

When I was not actually advising on set I did from time to time give medical advice to tide someone over until they were able to get to see their own doctor. Nobody took advantage of my presence, though, and it was not long before I found myself accepted as one of the extended *Dangerfield* family. This was in fact necessary if I was to do my job properly. In a very short time I had to learn the foibles and ways of the director, assistant directors, camera crew and, last but not least, the actors themselves. A good adviser must be able to stand and say nothing unless he is asked. They all know what they are doing but like to see him there so that instant help is at hand if necessary. True professionals that they were, they always asked before undertaking a medical procedure even though they had probably done it many times before, just to make sure that when the first assistant director shouted, 'Stand by … Take!' it was all correct.

Once the camera starts to roll it is a very expensive business to stop it, especially if something does not go as had been previously perfected at the immediate pre-take rehearsal. On one occasion my wife had joined me on set and was made very welcome by the actors and the director, who invited her to stand with me just behind his chair where she could see all the action in the making. A female actor playing the part of a patient on the doctor's couch kept having difficulty delivering her lines as they rehearsed ready for a take. My wife noticed that she seemed to be uncomfortable because the back of the couch was at a difficult angle for the 'patient' to talk and breathe easily. Assuming her customary wifely role as back seat driver, she whispered to me to raise the back of the couch. I duly passed this on to the director. Once this had been done there was no problem and we were able to go straight into a perfect take.

'Thank you, Doctor,' said the director, but without further ado I gave credit where it was due, and we both enjoyed watching the episode when it eventually reached our screen.

Sometimes I did find a tendency for 'patients' to overact and had to tell them gently to soft pedal it a bit, always afterwards reassuring them that their performance was exactly how a genuine patient would behave. Once or twice, however, realism went a little too far.

There was in one episode a scene where a dead body (actually a live extra) was laid waiting for Dangerfield to confirm death. At this stage the actress, who had been clad in a wet suit under her clothes, was having buckets of cold water poured over her to get the authentic drowned look when the camera zoomed in. There was a little delay in having to repeat the take, so after half an hour she was still lying there, having had many gallons of water poured on her. When the scene was eventually 'in the can' she was on the verge of hypothermia. Fortunately, the landlord of a nearby pub had offered his lounge as a green room so she was moved into a warm atmosphere at once. It nevertheless took about an hour before she was restored to normal.

For any event such as this I had to sign the official BBC accident book. This is kept for such eventualities by the second assistant director but fortunately very rarely used. His main function is to get the artists on set and then get

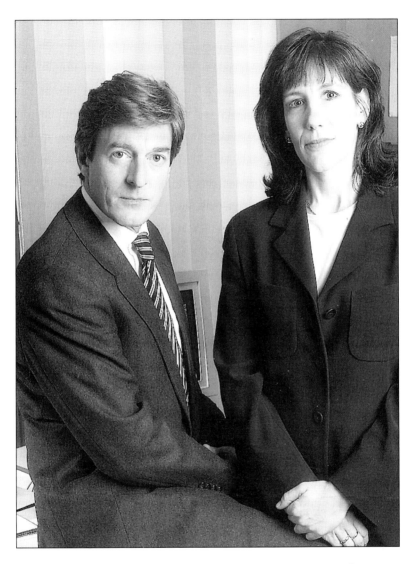

Nigel Havers as Dr Jonathan Paige in the fifth series, with Jane Gurnett as DI Gillian Cramer. (*BBC Picture Publicity*)

them to fill in their expenses forms before they go home. I gather there is usually no difficulty in fulfilling this part of his duties.

On another occasion, towards the end of the fourth series, the surgery was to be set on fire. As always the stuntmaster sent many hours preparing the stunt. The story called for a mentally disturbed woman to douse herself in petrol, then set light to herself and the petrol on the carpet. The firemen were all in position to douse the flames as soon as the camera had it in the can. There would be no second take on this one.

Together with two paramedics in flameproof overalls, I was stationed by the stuntmaster in a strategic position at the side of the set in case we were needed. Fortunately, we were not, but it was a close run thing and certainly illustrated that even the best laid plans can go wrong.

The conflagration took hold quickly, but suddenly there was a loud bang and a flash. The fire crew did their job well, if a little earlier than expected. The lady doing the stunt was singed but otherwise unharmed, thanks to the special fireproof clothing she had next to her skin and the insulation procedures she and her dressers had carried out beforehand. She was shaken, but ready to do another take if needed!

The stuntmaster was singed markedly over his hair and eyebrows and his face was red all over. I thought the skin would blister and peel off but a liberal application of flamazine cream by one of the paramedics stopped the burning sensation in the skin, which after three hours was back to its normal appearance although the singed hair would remain until it was combed out. These stunt people certainly earn their fee.

One of my most pleasant duties as medical adviser was the close working relationship I had with the make-up department. Helen, Vicky, Jane and Sarah not only made

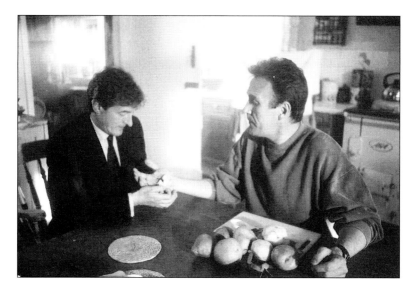

Nigel Havers, with Joe McGann, illustrating that it is often the smallest of cuts that tells so much – another triumph for the make-up department! (*BBC Picture Publicity*)

the best cup of coffee on the campus but in their comfortable caravan patiently and efficiently went about their work dealing in the most sympathetic way with the moods of the various actors. Even the best are nervous just before they go on camera and show it in different ways.

The make-up designer and her assistants were a sounding board for all, but with smiles and a few quiet words to their clients they would apply their various creams and potions from dawn to dusk. Everyone felt and looked better for their attention. The work having been completed, they would take a polaroid photograph of it, not for personal vanity but because every time an artist went on camera their appearance had to be the

111

same. Not a hair out of place even if the appearances may be hours, days, or even weeks apart.

My job was to advise them on the make-up for patients with different conditions and also, especially, different types of wounds. This I did by showing them police photographs and looking at their handiwork before they took the necessary photograph so that the wound could be rebuilt as often as the director wanted.

One day they had constructed a very life-like and graphic set of bruises on a baby that in the script had been fatally shaken when gripped around the chest, a not uncommon cause of death I had seen in dealing with child abuse cases. My co-adviser had in fact provided the original photographs and advised the team in matters of colouring and distribution of the bruises. The result of their handiwork was clearer than the original police photographs so Peter, who does a little teaching at detective training courses, showed the *Dangerfield* photos to his classes.

Of course, the experienced students recognised them as bruises caused in the manner alleged. But none would believe they were not genuine police prints and had been made from *Dangerfield* make-up department polaroid originals. Peter in his teaching now lays extra stress on the importance of proving in court the continuity of evidence. Barristers quite rightly are very particular about this, and this example illustrates the need to be so. Forensic evidence is being attacked more often in the courts following recent successful decisions in the Court of Appeal. If our make-up ladies could so convincingly create wounds, then the villains may also be able to use such techniques to pervert the course of justice. It has been an object lesson in the need to be ever vigilant in testing the forensic and photographic evidence, which in some cases in the past has been too readily accepted.

I have written about my time with *Dangerfield* at some length as the questions I am most often asked in my semi-retirement range from the cynical copper who asks, 'What's it like with the luvvies, Doctor?', to the police-women and secretaries who ask how they can get a job as an extra working with Pebble Mill's own police surgeon. Dr Dangerfield comes over as the perfect professional, the one that the viewer would love to have standing at the end of their bed if they were ill, but not so ill as to be unable to appreciate it! There have been many positive benefits from the programme in the health education field too, and a certain amount of accident prevention 'advice'. At last the public appreciates what the work of a police surgeon involves – and his family life, if a little unusual for the majority of my colleagues, has at least shown that doctors too have their problems.

At the time of writing, we have just finished filming the fifth series and as regular viewers know, our hero Paul Dangerfield has left the practice to take an academic post in a Department of Clinical Forensic Medicine at a prestigious university overseas.

His replacement partner Dr Jonathan Paige (played by Nigel Havers) has taken over and a few new faces have appeared among the police personnel.

The practice still carries on under the old name of Dangerfield, a not uncommon practice in country towns when the senior partner retires. The series also has retained its original name.

It may well be that Dr Paul, in the fullness of time, may tire of the academic life. Even plain homesickness may find him returning to his roots in Warwickshire. Who knows what the future holds?

Meanwhile, the new Dr Paige has settled in well and has dealt with some interesting and fascinating cases. His off duty relationships and social life provide an interesting

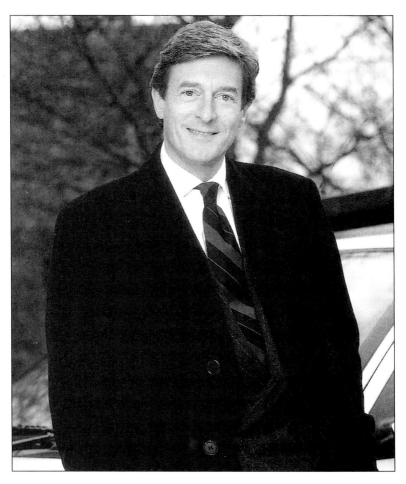

Nigel Havers in the new Dangerfield series (*BBC Picture Publicity*)

thread throughout the series which I am sure will lead to a great deal of interest and speculation for certain viewers! Just remember the old forensic aphorism 'Things are not always what they first seem'.

10

TIME
FOR A CHANGE

Retirement was not a word that featured in my vocabulary. During my days in general practice I had seen so many men retire after a busy working life and, after the initial period when they had done all those things they had promised themselves, go into a state of decline. The rate seemed to be in direct proportion to the amount of spare time that lay heavy on their hands.

I served with six Chief Constables and numerous assistants, and (much more important!) I had looked after, in quite a few instances, two generations of police officers where children had followed their parents into the force. The very last recruit I examined was Nicola Clarke on 20th December 1995. Her father Barry was one of the stalwarts of the Dog Section. He had unfortunately to be medically discharged after 27 years' service as a result of injuries received on duty.

I had been Nicola's doctor from birth and although a happy occasion to pass her fit to undertake the duties of a constable, it was also a poignant but appropriate moment to lay my stethoscope down for the last time in the service of the Northamptonshire Police.

As the new year broke I went straight into location work on the third series of *Dangerfield* and was still heavily committed with Presidential duties for the Association, so I did not really have any spare time on my hands. I even had to turn down increasing medico-legal work which I was being offered because I could not be sure I would be free from my BBC commitments to attend court if required. Attending evening classes in Italian was an absolute must as I was, after filming finished in May, due to visit my daughter in Rome and then spend some time in Tuscany. Therefore my time was fully taken up and the months passed quickly.

On my return from Italy, time started to drag and for a couple of weeks I found myself pushing trolleys around the supermarket, learning for the first time how much it actually costs to feed the family. Unfortunately, it did not provoke reactive anorexia as my wife hoped but it did stop me from questioning the housekeeping budget. Then there was a sudden change again in my fortunes, which came out of the blue.

The medical director of the Eastern Region of Her Majesty's Prison Service had heard of my relatively recent enforced idleness. He had a problem in that the practice that looked after HMP Wellingborough had given it up at the beginning of the year and, despite being well advertised, nobody had applied for the post. A locum medical officer had been used, but this was driving the budget right through the roof. So I was invited to help them out for just twelve hours a week for three months, and if I found it was not too onerous, perhaps a bit longer. From 1982 until 1992 I had been visiting medical officer to HMP Gartree when it was a Category A prison housing some of the most dangerous prisoners in the country.

I made a swift phone call to the practice that had done the job since it was a young offenders' prison some years ago. I found that it had now been reclassified as an adult prison Category C. As such it had about 100 lifers, who had all been inside for many years and were really no trouble as all they wanted was a quiet life with no hiccups to prevent them going out on parole at the earliest possible date. The other 200 prisoners were serving various sentences for all sorts of offences but it was estimated that 80 to 90 per cent of the crimes were drug related.

The other practice had found these prisoners very demanding and manipulative, but in view of my past experience at Gartree as well as with the police, their spokesman was confident that, 'You will soon sort them out, Hugh!'

Well, I did at least have plenty of time on my hands and could spend time talking, which I had found from my Gartree days was much more appreciated by the prisoner patients than just reaching out for the prescription pad. Quite a few ex-Gartree patients were waiting for me when I took up post, so my reputation (which was fortunately favourable) I found had gone before me on the prison grapevine. I must say I was most surprised how nearly all of them had matured in the few years since we had last met.

I might add that some of my prisoner patients in Gartree and more so in Wellingborough were found guilty partly on forensic evidence I had provided, but none of them bore me any malice or ill will. Many greeted me like an old friend and one of them expressed the view that 'it was better than the NHS as you do get continuity of care.'

I was surprised by the welcome they all gave me on my return to the prison service. Most of them claimed they were in my category of what I call 'honest crooks', who were only guests of Her Majesty because they had been defended by incompetent barristers or else had been 'stitched up' by the police. I remember a prison chaplain once made a remark to me to the effect that 'there is never a saint who has not been a sinner and never a sinner that cannot be redeemed.' I really believe that many of them have improved since they came into prison and are at last leading law-abiding and useful lives which hopefully they will continue on release.

I have been extremely fortunate in meeting many interesting people and making many friends in my career, first in my general practice and work in the local hospital, then in my forensic work. There I have been able to develop my interest in applying my medical knowledge to the law, not only to help bring guilty persons to justice, but also, and equally important, to ensure that the innocent are not wrongly arraigned.

As I look out of the window and see my daughter's sheep munching their hay I tell them to make it last. One thing is for certain, I can't afford any more hay! Those days have gone. But although never rich in the monetary sense, we have always lived in comfort and in good health – which, I can assure you, is more valuable than anything riches can ever buy.

ACKNOWLEDGEMENTS

I wish to express my grateful appreciation to the many people who have helped me, especially:

Pat Percival, Media and Public Relations Dept, Northamptonshire Police, for the idea and initial encouragement.

Peter Hall, Editor *Image* magazine, Northampton, alias 'Trotwood' in *Horse and Hound* magazine (and other country journals), for proof reading and corrections of which there were many.

Mark Edwards, Editor *Northampton Chronicle and Echo*, for his prompt response to my request for certain photographs and for permission to publish in the text. Also to Mrs Ros Spencer, librarian, for research and the provision of old press cuttings which were most useful for checking against my memory.

Rather than use recent police photographs, especially those that have not previously been in public domain, I felt some points in the text could be better illustrated by stills from *Dangerfield*, the BBC programme now in its fifth series. I am grateful for the help of Matthew Robinson and Stuart Humphreys of BBC Network Drama Publicity for their help in providing photographs and the permission to reproduce them.

Bob Thomas/Popperfoto photograph library, Overstone, Northampton for permission to use the photograph of Maurice Fitch.

Warwickshire Constabulary for their assistance and permission to use the photographs of Gordon Wardell.

A special thank you to former dog handler Brian Stockwin, who was responsible for superannuating Nero to Creaton House and also for finding some old photographs for me.

Nicholas Battle, my publisher of Countryside Books, who was at all times encouraging and supportive, enabling me to produce a coherent script from many pages of random and unnecessary verbosity.

Most of all, I thank all those men and women of the Northamptonshire Police with whom I worked for 37 years, sometimes at very unsociable hours and on some very unusual assignments. Amazingly, in all that time I cannot remember a cross word ever being spoken between us. There are not many jobs one can say that about! Thank you all – this is your story as much as it is mine.

INDEX

121